The Adventures of a Hypnotherapist

"Was I under?"

Also by Steve Burgess:

Famous Past Lives (O Books)
ISBN: 978 1 84694 494 9

The Power of Past Life Regression (6th Books)
ISBN: 978 1 78904 343 3

What People Are Saying About

The Adventures of a Hypnotherapist

Steve Burgess takes you on a fascinating journey in his book *The Adventures of a Hypnotherapist*. He is a great storyteller and shares many of the unusual case studies from his 30-year career as a Hypnotherapist. His love for his work and compassion for his clients shines through, and he is not afraid to go places with his clients that other therapists might shy away from including alien abductions, spirit attachments, and past life regression. His passion for past life regression is apparent throughout the book as he shares many of the amazing client transformations from receiving this powerful therapy; he truly is an expert in his field. This book will appeal to all kinds of therapists and those interested in the workings of our amazing unconscious minds.
Marcia Tillman MSc, hypnotherapist, hypnotherapy trainer, and founder of Life Clinics (UK) www.lifeclinics.com

Steve Burgess says he writes 'to entertain and not to educate', but I would totally disagree with him. He does write in a brilliantly entertaining and conversational way, but *The Adventures of a Hypnotherapist* will also educate a wide readership, i.e. many different professionals – not just hypnotherapists – and the lay person. The book presents Burgess' vast experience of being a hypnotherapist over three decades. The verbal accounts from actual (anonymised) clients are fascinating and detailed; and also cover a wide range of subjects – including abuse, witches, and satanic rings.
This book will challenge every reader – from the sceptic, to someone who is curious about hypnotherapy, regression therapy and past lives – and to the more experienced therapist. It makes you think and reflect, but also to question one's own beliefs, values and ways of living and working.

Burgess does give an insight into theory and techniques, but what is so refreshing is that he is honest about his thoughts and doubts which have arisen during practice.
Jacki Pritchard, clinical hypnotherapist, independent social worker, and author of *Hypnotherapy for Pregnancy and Birthing, Hypnotherapy Scripts to Promote Children's Well-being,* and *Dealing with Different Types of Losses Using Hypnotherapy Scripts.* Jacki Pritchard Ltd., www.jp-hypnotherapy.co.uk and www.jackipritchard.co.uk

This book is an excellent adventure into Past Life Therapy, authored by, in my opinion, my 'go-to' expert in this field. People question such 'Woo-woo' methods, however reading this book the evidence is evident that 'something' is happening for these amazing changes to people's lives, once they have experienced these techniques. The book is an easy and absorbing narrative to read, peppered with other blended techniques, to keep you wanting to learn more. The book is sprinkled also with Steve's humour, which lightens what could be perceived as a heavy topic. I highly recommend this book.
Kevin Laye, founder of PsyTap

I've loved reading *The Adventures of a Hypnotherapist;* in fact, I couldn't put the book down! It was fascinating to embark on a journey with such varied and unusual cases.
I became intrigued to discover what happened to each client as they took courageous steps toward their transformation and healing.
Sometimes I was in stitches laughing at Steve's unique wit and humour — especially when the content reminded me of similar incidents from my own practice!
I really felt I was in a front row seat in his office, as Steve expertly dealt with very sensitive problems and delicate issues in a compassionate manner.

I wholeheartedly recommend this book to anyone who is curious, has an interest in Hypnosis or is studying Hypnotherapy. There is so much to learn from the way Steve handles individual cases with flexibility, compassion, insight and wisdom.
Michelle A. Hardwick, hypnotherapist, retreat facilitator, and QHHT practitioner, www.michellehardwick.com

The Adventures of a Hypnotherapist takes readers on an intriguing journey into the realms of the unconscious mind, through a fascinating collection of case studies. The author has many years of experience with regression of all kinds and takes readers into past lives, alien abductions, and ancestral journeys with a sure hand. He showcases the profound impact these experiences have had on the lives of his clients, and how releasing trauma is the key to personal growth and emotional freedom.
The stories give a real insight into not just the author's intriguing work, but also his skill, compassion and empathy, which shine through on every page.
The Adventures of a Hypnotherapist is essential reading for anyone keen to explore the mysteries of the mind and the soul.
Debbie Waller, therapist and founder and principal of Yorkshire Hypnotherapy Training

I've had the pleasure of knowing Steve Burgess for the last 15 years, closely witnessing his remarkable ability to captivate his audience and students. His unique teaching style and storytelling prowess, coupled with his skill in addressing the root causes of people's issues, stand out distinctly. As a colleague in the field of hypnotherapy and regression, I can conclude his depth of knowledge, experience, and genuine care for others are unparalleled. These qualities shine through in *The Adventures of a Hypnotherapist*.
In this book, Steve artfully explains the innate power we possess to heal psychological and physical issues by addressing

emotional wounds, as well as harnessing the mind's natural ability to do amazing things like anaesthetise the body before surgery. He masterfully intertwines factual information, client anecdotes, and his own challenges and triumphs, and he does so with sincerity and humour, making the book highly entertaining, captivating and enlightening.

I wholeheartedly recommend this book to anyone interested in personal and spiritual growth, the interplay between mind, body, and soul, and the transformative power of past life regression and hypnotherapy. Guided by Steve's expert narrative craft, this book promises an unforgettable journey.

Kenneth Soares, hypnotherapist, speaker, and co-founder of Power Thoughts Meditation Club

The Adventures of a Hypnotherapist

"Was I Under?"

by

Steve Burgess

BOOKS
London, UK
Washington, DC, USA

CollectiveInk

First published by O-Books, 2025
O-Books is an imprint of Collective Ink Ltd.,
Unit 11, Shepperton House, 89 Shepperton Road, London, N1 3DF
office@collectiveinkbooks.com
www.collectiveinkbooks.com
www.o-books.com

For distributor details and how to order please visit the 'Ordering' section on our website.

ISBN: 978 1 80341 805 6
978 1 80341 813 1 (ebook)
Library of Congress Control Number: 2024933765

A CIP catalogue record for this book is available from the British Library.

Design: Lapiz Digital Services

To my Team with great affection; you are my legacy

Contents

Acknowledgements

Being a Hypnotherapist is not an easy job; day after day hearing our clients' stories which are sometimes harrowing in the extreme, and then holding the space and guiding each client to a (hopefully) successful resolution of their issues. It takes determination, stamina, and an open heart to work in this way, but having good therapy techniques can make all the difference to success in our client work. I've been fortunate to have had training from three men whom I consider to have made a significant impact on my journey as a therapist. Firstly, Wilf Proudfoot, who inspired many of my colleagues and myself to work with the client's inner process to facilitate change. As Wilf's dear friend, Virginia Satir, wrote about the therapy process — 'I own me. Therefore, I can engineer me'. Secondly, Ernest Rossi, the brilliant Hypnotherapist/psychotherapist who was the primary acolyte of Milton Erickson for the final eight years of Erickson's life, who taught me that it's vitally important to trust the client's subconscious and to get out of the way whilst it helps the client to heal. Thirdly, Gary Craig, the creator of EFT and who (despite only claiming to be an engineer) is one of the finest therapists I have ever seen.

Of course, I have also learnt much along the way from many colleagues in the profession, and am grateful for their kindness in sharing wisdom as I grew from being a 'rookie therapist' to a 'jobbing therapist', which I still simply class myself as even after three decades of doing 'The Work'.

With regards to this book, several people are owed big thanks from me for their guidance and assistance. Firstly, my friend John Crick in Missouri in the USA; his advice on what to throw out and what to amend in the first draft of the book was so helpful. Then, thanks to those who proofread the manuscript — my dad (who also came up with the sub-title 'Was I Under?'), and my friend, Vicki Howd.

I give special thanks to my team member, Monique Glover, whose thoughts and suggestions at critical points along the writing process were invaluable; not only is she a terrific Hypnotherapist but she's also a creative genius.

I also pay credit to all of my team members for their loyalty to me and more particularly for their dedication to their clients and their passion for regression therapy – Fil Woodhouse, Michael Hearn and Monique Glover; each of you is an inspiration.

And finally, ever grateful thanks to all of my clients over the years, from whom I learnt so much and without whom this book would not have been possible.

Prologue

'...Tell them, that, to ease them of their griefs,
Their fears of hostile strokes, their aches, losses,
Their pangs of love, with other incident throes
That nature's fragile vessel doth sustain
In life's uncertain voyage, I will some kindness
do them.'

Timon of Athens
Shakespeare and Middleton

This book is not an academic textbook from which you'll learn a lot of information about how to use hypnosis or how to become a Hypnotherapist. It may be a manifesto for the power of hypnotherapy, but above all it's simply a record of some of the more unusual experiences of my career and some of the most interesting of the more than 15,000 therapy sessions that I have facilitated. I write to entertain and not to educate. I hope you enjoy the stories that I tell, and if you learn something along the way, it will be by accident and not design. As one of my favourite writers, Jerome K Jerome, wrote in 1886 in the preface to *The Idle Thoughts of an Idle Fellow*:

> 'I have ventured to offer these mere "idle thoughts" of mine as mental food for the English-speaking peoples of the earth. What readers ask nowadays in a book is that it should improve, instruct, and elevate. This book wouldn't elevate a cow. I cannot conscientiously recommend it for any useful purposes whatever.'

All of the stories herein are true, with no fabrication in any way. At the risk of appearing to only use regression into past lives and not into this life, even though a great deal of my work involves healing emotional wounds from childhood in this present life, I have deliberately not written much about my client's traumas that have taken place in their present lives but have chosen to focus mainly on their experiences from previous lifetimes. There are a few reasons for this. Firstly, past life regression is fascinating. I think your jaw will drop when you read the incredible variety of past life stories and the wide range of issues that can be healed using Past Life Therapy. Secondly, I feel that writing about my client's present lives traumas (many of which were in their childhoods) may be a little too intrusive, whereas past life traumas seem to be less immediate and one step removed from them. Thirdly, I want to highlight how effective it is as a therapeutic process. I am tired of people who mock it without investigating it in depth.

I realise that some of the things I write about, and some of my viewpoints, will be controversial, and you may find it difficult to believe my claims and assertions. But, dear reader, all I ask is that you keep an open, inquiring mind and that you remember that the mind is like a parachute — it works best when it is open.

I'll begin by sharing with you one of the more sensational cases from my 30-year professional career, before we move into other aspects of the fascinating world of hypnotherapy and my life as a Hypnotherapist.

Please note that all of my clients' names have been changed in order to ensure confidentiality.

Trigger Warning: Some chapters contain material related to rape and sexual abuse in therapy sessions; if you're likely to find this unpleasant or triggering please do not read on.

Chapter 1

Face to Face with a Death Sentence

Early in 1994 a new client with a life-threatening illness turned up at my consulting rooms desperate for help. Emma, an attractive woman in her early 30s, had to be helped up the stairs to my office by her mother and a friend. She was so thin that she looked like a human stick insect. She flopped down in the reclining chair that I used for hypnosis sessions and told me that she had been given 6 months to live by her specialist at the local hospital. She was suffering from a rare disease called Focal Nodular Hyperplasia (no, I'd never heard of it either until that day). Focal Nodular Hyperplasia is a disease in which non-cancerous tumours grow on the liver. Emma's FNH was unusually aggressive in that the tumours were growing rapidly. The resulting pain, not just from the diseased liver but particularly from the pressure that the tumours were placing upon her internal organs, was immense. She was in agony most of the time and doped up to the eyeballs on morphine. This meant that she hardly knew which day of the week it was (a Tuesday, actually, though why you need to know that is beyond me). She had experienced surgery twice as the medics tried to help her; both times disastrously.

Emma lived alone with her 5-year-old daughter, but for the past few months she had been unable to look after her daughter or spend quality time with her because of the chronic pain she was suffering from. She was highly allergic to painkillers, so much so that just one aspirin could kill her (I told her not to take any in that case, just to be on the safe side!). She was so ill that she spent most of each day lying in pain on her bed. She had no appetite as she felt sick most of the time (if she did eat, she would often vomit it back up again) resulting in a significant loss of weight. In the weight loss world this is known as the 'near death diet' and is not a diet usually recommended by Weight Watchers.

Emma sat in front of me in a daze, lines of pain on her face and on the verge of tears. She felt exhausted by the battle to survive, by the constant, debilitating pain, and by the side effects of the various drugs that she had been given by her doctor and the specialists at the hospital.

My heart went out to her as I listened to her story. She had almost lost all hope that she could survive the illness. The unremitting pain was dragging her down and the National Health Service Consultant assigned to her had completely given up on her. It was he who had pronounced her death sentence, giving her no more than 6 months to live. With a look of unbearable sadness on her face she told me 'You're my final resort, my last hope'. So, no pressure there then!

I wondered just how could I help her? Yes, I knew the amazing power of the subconscious mind. Also, I had often read of people who were close to death suffering from apparently incurable illnesses and who had been given up on by their doctors. Somehow, they had found the miracle that they were looking for and come back to health again. Sometimes they had visited a healer or a complementary therapist and had been healed of their complaint. Sometimes they had changed their lifestyle or their diet, or found that affirmations or meditation had brought them back to life again. I had read of one woman who had only a short time to live as most of her internal organs had stopped working; she had begun sending love over and over to every organ in her body and over time she recovered and was completely well again.

But here I was face to face with a human being who was clearly on the downward slope and who might not survive the walk back down my stairs at the end of our appointment, let alone get through the next few weeks. I felt completely daunted by the challenge. Did I seriously think that I could help her? And what if I couldn't? Here was a massively serious situation, quite unlike anything I had been faced with during my previous two years as a Hypnotherapist.

I was used to treating traumas, phobias and anxiety, helping people to stop smoking and lose weight, but nothing as serious as this. I was well-trained and had done a lot of research into different ways of using hypnosis, so I knew the theory of what could help Emma, but knowing theory and putting it into practice in real life are two entirely different things. Something inside me, though, drove me on to accept the challenge. It may have been that I was subconsciously playing out some archetypal knight in shining armour rescues damsel-in-distress role, or it may have been that I was over-confident in my abilities as a therapist, but I prefer to believe that it was my Higher Self, my subconscious mind, that already knew that working with Emma was the right thing to do. Having facilitated so many thousands of therapy sessions, I now know from experience that the subconscious often knows what is going to happen to us in advance of it happening. Before I continue with Emma's story, let me share with you an example of this phenomena.

The 'father' of modern-day hypnotherapy was called Milton Erickson. An American psychiatrist, he became interested in hypnosis and subsequently used hypnotherapy with many of his patients, in incredibly creative ways. He always believed that his patient's subconscious knew best and he revolutionised the way in which hypnotherapy was used. An example of the way in which the subconscious knows the future is exemplified by the time when Erickson was demonstrating a therapy technique known as 'Automatic Writing' to a psychology department at an American university.

With this technique, the hypnotised person is told that they will open their eyes and write something on a piece of paper. They don't have to know what it is they are writing but they will find a word or some words will just come into their mind all by themselves when they are given a piece of paper and a pen by the therapist. They are then instructed to open their eyes and are given paper and a pen. They write a word or some words down, give the paper and pen back to the therapist, close their eyes and go back into hypnosis. The technique can be used to uncover a clue or to gain some insights that can be used to resolve the problem that they are working on in therapy. When they come out of trance at the end of the session they may or may not remember writing the words.

In this case, Erickson demonstrated on a lady called Peggy. In front of a group of students he took her into trance, gave her suggestions that she would write something on a piece of paper and then go back into trance. She did this, but once she had written something she automatically folded the piece of paper up and put it in her bag. Then she closed her eyes and went back into trance. Later, when he brought her out of hypnosis, Erickson didn't mention anything about this to her, she didn't talk about it, and she left with everyone else at the end of the meeting. This was in April.

Five months later, in September, Peggy called him at his office, saying that she had found a piece of paper in her bag and she thought that Erickson was in some way connected with it. She didn't know how the paper got there, but on it (in strange handwriting) was written the words 'Will I marry Harold?'

Erickson confessed that it was something to do with his lecture several months earlier at the university. He asked her if, at the time of his lecture, she was engaged to anyone and she said that she was, but that she was engaged to Bill. He questioned her further and she told him that in April she had no doubts about her engagement to Bill, but then in June she and Bill broke up and in July she got married to a man called Harold!

In April she had only seen Harold at the university, but she had never met him or talked to him. She only knew him by sight.

Her subconscious already knew that she was going to break up with Bill because Harold was the man who truly appealed to her. Erickson felt that the reason that she'd folded the piece of paper up and put it into her bag was that consciously she couldn't stand facing that fact in April. But the amazing fact was that her subconscious already knew what was going to happen.

So, call it gut instinct or intuition, but my subconscious pushed me into working with Emma, when it would have been easier for me to have turned her down because of the severity of her problem. And I am so glad that I did because it soon transpired that I had two aces up my sleeve. Firstly, Emma was a fighter, with oceans of courage and the determination to beat the illness. Secondly, she was good in trance. This means that she had a natural ability to go into hypnosis, which meant that from our very first hypnosis session her subconscious mind was able to do the work that we needed to do, and to do it effectively.

When she was ready to go into hypnosis, I asked Emma to gaze on her fingers and I gave her suggestions that her eyelids would start to feel heavy. Within a short time her eyes were closed and she was laid in my reclining chair in a state of deep relaxation. Her breathing was calm and regular, her body was supine and quite still. The speed with which she went into trance told me that she was one of the 25–30% of people who are naturally hypnotic (I call them 'Number Ones', for reasons which I'll explain later). This meant that it was easy for her to enter a state of hypnosis and that she would be able to tap into the power of her subconscious mind in a deeper way than most people. I knew then that we had a good chance of working together to help her to stay alive.

In that first session I simply took Emma into trance and gave her post-hypnotic suggestions that after the session she would feel calm and at peace, that her subconscious would help her to let go of the pain, and that her body and mind would work together to help her to heal. Most importantly, I also asked her to visualise herself completely healed; to run a movie in her mind of how she wanted to be in the future, and to experience the feelings of how that would feel. This type of visualisation, called Positive Future Image Rehearsal (also known as Future Pacing), plants a seed of wellness in the subconscious and gives it something to work towards. If a person keeps imagining themselves how they want to be in the future, and if they regularly experience the feelings of how they want to be, their subconscious will create a journey to take them into that future state. Nowadays this concept has been popularised by the book and the movie *The Secret*.

When Emma came out of trance, she looked so different to how she had looked 30 minutes earlier. She looked lighter and she told me that she felt calmer than she had felt for months. She also felt optimistic that hypnotherapy might help her. I gave her one of my hypnotherapy recordings to play at home, she made an appointment to see me a week later and she departed, able to walk back down the stairs unaided.

Chapter 2

Once Upon a Time…

When Emma returned for her next appointment she looked quite different — she no longer looked so drained and exhausted. She told me that the excruciating pain in her liver and abdomen had subsided substantially and that she had stopped taking the morphine; the benefits of this were that she felt much more clear-headed and able to start thinking and moving her body more. She was no longer spending most of each day lying in bed in pain. She knew she wasn't cured, but she felt that she was beginning to get her life back. It was a good start to her journey of healing.

I gave Emma an overview of the therapy process that we would be undertaking. Our sessions together would consist of standard hypnotherapy pain management techniques as well as visualisations in which she would imagine her body healing. We would use hypnotic suggestions too so that the subconscious mind would become programmed to heal the body. Most importantly we would also work on the *emotional* causes of the liver disease.

I realise that you may be sceptical when you read this, but my mind-world when it comes to sickness and physical problems (based not on a whim but on my experience of over 30 years as a therapist, working with the power of the mind) is that the vast majority of illness is caused by underlying negative emotions and energies that are locked inside a person. There are five negative emotions: anger, sadness, fear, anxiety and guilt. These emotions arise as a result of traumas and significant emotional events that have taken place in the past in this present lifetime, in previous lives, and in the lives of ancestors in our bloodline (parents, grandparents, great-grandparents etc., etc.).

We all have an emotional 'pressure cooker' in our minds and whenever we are traumatised by something it's as if we take the lid off the pressure cooker and put the negative emotions from the trauma into it. As we go through life and more traumas occur in our lives, we continue to take the lid off and fill up the pressure cooker. The pressure in it then builds up and we react to the pressure by suffering from anxiety, depression, phobias, illness etc.

I realise that this goes against the standard medical model which believes that an illness is something that a person catches for no apparent reason or because of lifestyle choices (poor diet, smoking etc.), but the modern medical model seems to be all about putting medicines inside people in order to make money for pharmaceutical companies. The concept of illness being caused by emotions has been eloquently advocated by Louise Hay in her wonderful book *You Can Heal Your Life*. She herself claimed to have cured her own breast cancer by working on its emotional causes and by using affirmations and visualisations to heal herself; I'll write more about working with cancer later in this book.

The aim of regression therapy is to travel back in trance to the emotional root causes of the illness, wherever the traumas have taken place (in this life, past lives or our ancestor's lives), in order to re-experience the traumas and to let go of the emotions and energies that got locked inside the subconscious mind. It isn't a fun process, and usually we see a lot of tears in a regression session, but it is the most powerful form of therapy that I know. My book *The Power of Past Life Regression* documents in more depth the effectiveness of this therapy.

Once we had finished discussing the treatment protocol, I guided Emma into trance, talking quietly and gently about her body and mind relaxing. Her eyelids closed, her body softened, her breathing slowed down and she lay in my reclining chair looking very peaceful.

When I work in regression I use a technique called an Ideo-Motor Response (IMR). Through the use of the IMR, rather than me telling the client where we have to go to uncover the traumas, the client's subconscious itself leads the way. Once Emma was in a pleasant state of hypnosis, I asked her subconscious to take control of one of her fingers on her non-dominant hand, by making one of her fingers feel very, very light. As I continued talking in this way, giving suggestions for a finger to feel weightless like a helium-filled balloon, sure enough after a couple of minutes her index finger started to slowly rise up into the air. I could see the look of surprise on Emma's face as this happened. She knew that she wasn't moving her finger consciously; it was floating in the air all by itself. This Ideo-Motor Response meant that her subconscious mind was now in control of her finger. I asked her subconscious to use the finger to signal 'yes' and 'no' to my questions by floating the finger up into the air to signal 'yes', and to keep the finger resting in a stationery position to signal 'no'. I then asked the subconscious to let the finger float back down again. As it did so, Emma sighed and went deeper into trance.

I then asked her subconscious to focus on the emotional causes of her liver disease, and to indicate (using the IMR finger) whereabouts in the past significant emotional events or traumas had taken place which were connected to causing her illness. I asked firstly if there were any events in this lifetime — it responded by raising the finger to signal 'yes'. I asked if there were any past life causes — again the finger rose to signal 'yes'. It answered 'no' to the question of any inherited traumas from her ancestors. We now knew where we had to regress to, in order to release the locked-in emotions that were causing the Focal Nodular Hyperplasia.

Thus began Emma's entry into the world of hypnotherapy. Over the next few months she experienced many hypnotherapy sessions. In some of them, she experienced healing visualisations and post-hypnotic suggestions which I gave her so that her subconscious mind was programmed to use its power to heal her physical body and to create a positive outcome. She also used pain reduction techniques and self-hypnosis to make sure the pain levels were under control. She visualised the tumours shrinking and her liver healing. We regressed into childhood and did work to heal her Inner Child. Two of her past lives were interesting; in one of them she was a Native American woman killed by another tribe which was raiding her village. She was grabbed from behind and stabbed. Guess where the knife went? Straight through her lower back and into her liver.

In the second past life she was a young man murdered in WWII. The exact details were sketchy but during a skirmish he fell into a river and was bayoneted. Once more, the blade went into the young man's back and liver, killing him. His body was left to float downstream by the killers. In both regressions she experienced a lot of fear and then total relief after she had died and her spirit had left her body.

If you are new to this concept of Past Life Therapy then all of this possibly appears to be fantastical. However, it is standard fare for a past life regression session. Remember, the regression 'model' is that all of our issues as human beings come from locked-in feelings and emotions from past traumas. Once we regress back into the traumas and release the locked-in feelings and emotions, the problems that they are causing get better — sometimes miraculously so. At a risk of sounding as if I'm trying to flog you my previous book, if you want to get more of a handle on the subject of past life regression read *The Power of Past Life Regression*.

Over time, as a result of our sessions, Emma began to get better. Her pain was substantially reduced, her weight improved as she was able to eat more, and she was able to start living a more normal life. She felt, for the first time in a long time, some hope that she could beat this illness. She told me that she felt that she was starting to get her life back. Her medical specialists were amazed that the tumours had stopped growing and some were shrinking (although doubtless they just thought that this happened spontaneously for no apparent reason).

In one of our sessions that took place early on in the process, when she was in trance, I told her a story. This is called Metaphor Therapy and was pioneered by Milton Erickson, whom I mentioned earlier. Metaphors are an extremely powerful way to create change in a person, and I use them often with my clients. The subconscious loves metaphors, and I think we all do too as human beings. Even though my clients may be middle-aged or older, there is still a child part of them that loves listening to a story being told. I think this is a universalism — something that we can all connect with.

A metaphor is a story that symbolises the clients' problem and the resolution of that problem. Metaphors communicate indirectly, in that telling a story distracts the conscious mind and activates an unconscious search for meaning and resources. As such it is an excellent way of communicating with someone whilst they are in trance. The metaphor resonates in the subconscious and mobilises the resources needed to resolve the issue. The story line beguiles the conscious, left-brain mind and the unconscious gets the message and starts to make the necessary changes.

A metaphor will be a story of a journey from a client's present state to a desired state. Fairy tales are metaphors: 'Once upon a time' (present state) ... 'and they lived happily ever after' (desired state). Metaphors are often also reframing devices: an ugly duckling is really a beautiful swan. To this day, Emma still remembers the night that I told her a story as part of her healing journey. This is the story I told her:

> Once upon a time there was a little girl, and one day, when she was feeling very upset about some things in

her life, she went for a walk. Without realising where she was going, because she was feeling so bothered by things, she found herself walking into a forest. At first, she felt OK being there as it was such a nice place, but quite soon she realised that she couldn't find the way back out of the forest. She started to feel a little bit scared, but as she went on trying to find her way out, she found that she was going deeper and deeper into the forest, and the trees became thicker and the light grew dimmer; she knew that she was completely lost. She was lost and alone in the centre of a deep, dark wood. As she looked around the trees looked angry, the wind began to blow the branches and she could hear the loud rustling of the leaves. Through the branches she could see the sky was starting to darken, and she felt so scared that she wondered if she'd ever find her way back out to safety. She sat down and began to cry. It was as if everything was against her and she felt deeply unhappy, as if there was no way out and no way back to happiness. She could feel her body feeling tense and sick and panicky; her breathing was short and fast; she wondered if she was going to survive this. This went on for some time, with the light in the wood getting more and more gloomy and the wind whipping through the branches of the trees. She felt exhausted and was thinking about giving up. How could she find a way out? She felt that there was no way out, and that she'd be lost and alone here for ever. And then…

I don't know if you know this but sometimes, just when we feel that we're about to give up, as if we can't go on any longer, something changes inside us and something magical happens. And you do know that magic can happen, don't you?

Just as this little girl was about to give up, feeling that she couldn't go on any longer, she looked up and noticed a light that was beginning to shine in front of a tree just close to her. As she watched, this light began to grow stronger and stronger and bigger and bigger. It began to shine brightly and she could see that it was magically starting to form the shape of a person, the shape of someone dressed like a wizard. She watched in amazement as the light turned into a wise old wizard, who was then surrounded by a gentle light. At first the girl was unsure how to feel about this, but when the wizard smiled at her she began to relax and feel better. 'I think you're lost' said the wizard kindly. 'Maybe I can help you to find a way out of this dark place.' The wizard took the girl's hand and helped her to stand up. 'Look over here', he said gently, 'I think you'll notice there is a way out.' The girl looked to where the wizard was pointing, and with the help of the light shining around the wizard she saw that there was indeed a path. She hadn't spotted it before because she was too scared and panicky and feeling too sick, but now with the aid of the wizard's light she could see that there was a way out. 'Come with me, we'll walk together for a while', said the wizard, and the girl immediately started to feel better, knowing that she was no longer alone and that someone was going to help her. So, they walked hand in hand along the path, and as they did, quite magically the stormy weather started to ease down and the woodland began to be lighter and brighter. They walked hand in hand through the trees, along a different path than the one the girl had used earlier. She began to feel much calmer and much more confident that she was going to get out of the forest. She knew that she didn't have to find her own way out, but just trust that everything was going to be alright. As they walked, she could feel the wizard's energy was helping her to heal, and she could sense a feeling of strength growing inside her which she hadn't felt before. She didn't know where this inner strength came from, and when she asked the wizard about it, she was told that the inner strength had always been there, it was just that it hadn't been released in this way before. The girl felt very happy. As they came towards the edge of the trees, the girl felt so excited that she was free and had found her way out of the forest that she let go of the wizard's hand and ran forward out of the trees. She found herself in golden sunlight and she knew that from here she could find her way home. Excitedly, she turned to thank the wizard but found that the wizard was no longer there. He had helped the girl to find her way out of the darkness into the light and his work was now done. The girl stopped for a moment and then breathed deeply and smiled. She knew that she didn't need the wizard anymore, that she was OK on her own. She now felt much safer and stronger, and in some way she felt that she'd learnt something about herself because of this experience. She'd learnt that she did have all of the strength she needed to get through things. That although she'd had a bad time, she had come through it, as nothing lasts forever. She had survived. I wonder if you think she'd learnt anything else?

The girl was happy and healed, she ran home excitedly, looking forward to a new way of life.

Chapter 3

Hypno-Surgery (or How I Learn the Hard Way That Having a Phobia of Blood Is Not a Good Thing to Have in an Operating Theatre)

After several months of intensive therapy, Emma arrived for another session. As she sat in front of me, she told me that she had had an appointment with her Consultant at the hospital. The Consultant wanted to perform surgery on her again; the same surgery that she'd had twice before with appalling results. He felt that as she was now so much improved, she had a better chance of coming through the operation, which would obviously be an arduous experience for her.

The aim of the surgical procedure was to make a cut into the groin and insert a thin plastic tube through the incision, up into the veins and arteries that ran from her groin to her liver. Once the tube reached the liver, he would try to insert coils through it. The idea behind this is that the coils would attach themselves to the tumours and then cut off the blood supply to them, thus stopping them from growing and possibly even starving them to death.

Emma shared with me that she was highly allergic to anaesthetics. To complicate matters further, she was also allergic to the chemicals in a dye that she had to drink before surgery. As a result of these two allergies, Emma was fully awake during the previous two surgeries. She spent the whole procedure on the operating table retching and vomiting and in acute pain. The surgeon, who was trying to perform an extremely delicate procedure, had a hell of a time. While he was trying to thread the plastic tube up through her veins, Emma was jerking around and retching so much that not only did the surgery fail but he accidentally inflicted further damage on her already weakened body. Both times the operation had taken around two and a half hours, and both times afterwards she was in hospital for several weeks. The first time her gall bladder was so damaged that it had to be removed, the second time the liver itself was damaged.

Quite obviously Emma was worried about having to go through such a traumatic experience once more; she remembered only too well the pain and unpleasantness of it all. Yes, she was a brave woman (who deserves a medal for all that she has been through) but there's only so much that someone with a warrior spirit can take.

I can still remember sitting there that morning, listening to her explain all of this, and when she paused at the end of her story, I heard a voice saying these words to her: 'we'll do the operation in hypnosis'.

I looked around to see who had said them. Then I realised that the words had come out of my mouth. I don't know who was more shocked — me or Emma. But before I had chance to retract them, a bright smile lit up her face. 'Really', she said, smiling, 'that's fantastic, thank you. I'll check with the surgeon and see what he says.'

With a confused look on my face and a half-smile as if it was all OK, I just nodded. I now had to give the impression that this was an every-day occurrence in the life of a Hypnotherapist. 'What do I do now?' I asked myself.

I spent the next few days worrying about the possible consequences of what I had said, or maybe I should phrase that as what my *subconscious* had said. It had to have been my subconscious that made me speak those words, as my conscious mind knew that I hadn't been trained in hypno-surgery. In fact, to my knowledge, at that time in the UK no-one had been trained in it; I was opening myself up to one heck of a risk. I was hoping that Emma's surgeon would turn down the opportunity to take part in such an unusual venture, but to my surprise he agreed to it. I think that he had been so traumatised by the previous two attempts that he was prepared to try almost anything which would make his job easier. The date was arranged for the operation at the local infirmary (a Monday morning at 9.30 a.m.) and Emma felt a big relief because she believed that it was going to work. At least she was happy; I just felt the pressure of the awesome responsibility that was now resting on my shoulders to make sure that it would all go smoothly.

However, I did my research into using hypnosis in surgery and I insisted to Emma that we had plenty of practice sessions in advance of the big day to rehearse the processes that would be required in the operating theatre: to go into trance quickly and to anaesthetise her body so that she could experience the actual surgery without any pain and to stay in a calm state throughout the procedure. These sessions went very well and Emma felt confident that she could have the surgery and feel nothing apart from an inner peace. I just drank vodka every evening and prayed that it would all be OK.

One of the techniques I used is based on the methods of the Spanish surgeon, Dr Angel Escudero. He has performed over 10,000 surgical interventions (many of them involving major surgery) without ANY anaesthetic. He was featured in a BBC documentary called *Your Life in Their Hands* in which, amongst other things, he was filmed doing a major operation on his sister to straighten her right leg. Whilst she lies on the operating table, her leg is cut into and a deep incision made into the knee. Parts of the bone are then chiselled out using a hammer and chisel as well as a circular saw. An electric drill is then used to drill all the way through her calf and then all the way through her thigh so that steel rods can be inserted through the holes to keep the newly straightened leg in place. The surgery itself is conventional. What is not conventional is that the patient had no form of chemical painkiller and she spent the entire operation on her back completely aware of everything that was happening but without any pain! I have used Escudero's methods in conjunction with hypnosis many times over the years to help clients suffering from pain, sometimes with miraculous results.

Our rehearsals went well, and Emma was able to anaesthetise her body quite quickly and to maintain the analgesic state for an hour or two. I didn't know how long the actual surgery would take but I guessed that this would give the surgeon enough time to do what he had to do.

As the day of the operation drew closer, I become more nervous. I knew that there were so many things that could go wrong during the surgery. What if Emma was so nervous that she couldn't let herself go into trance? What if the psychological anaesthesia didn't work or it wore off halfway through the operation? What if she was constantly nauseous and retching throughout the procedure? This was a bloody serious situation I had got myself into, and the pressure was all on me to make sure that it all went as smoothly as possible. I told Emma that I was happy to meet the surgeon in advance of the big day in order to explain to him something of the nature of hypnosis and the methods I would be using, so that he could reassure himself that I knew what I was doing. He could then ask me any questions so that on the day we worked as a team to make sure we got Emma through it as smoothly as possible. She spoke to him but the only message I got back was to be at the hospital thirty minutes before the scheduled time of the operation.

Finally, the big day arrived and at 9 a.m. I presented myself to the surgical team at the hospital. There then followed a desperate search with the surgeon through locker rooms to furnish me with surgical clothing – trousers and gown, hat and shoes. It was all a bit chaotic and did nothing to calm my nerves. Finally, wearing all of the right gear but in all the wrong sizes, I scrubbed up and was taken through to the theatre. Picture the scene: Emma was already there, lying on the operating table. The periphery of the room was darkened whilst lights shone down onto her, and I could smell the strong smell of hospital cleaning products. Around her stood the surgical team and the surgeon. The consultant anaesthetist stood with her arms folded and a face like a slapped arse. She was not impressed that this bearded charlatan was making her redundant. I did my best to enter the room with authority, but the over-sized hat was slipping down over my eyes, the trousers were starting to fall down around my waist and the over-sized shoes were slopping around and making me walk like a drunken sailor. The too-small surgical shirt meant that I could hardly use my arms as to do so would possibly have torn it in two – I held them helplessly in front of me like a T-Rex. I looked like a cross between Norman Wisdom and Mr Blobby. The anaesthetist was beaming malice at me from her eyes, willing me to fail so she could jump in and save the situation when it was all going wrong. With as much dignity as I could muster (which was very little) I looked at the surgeon.

'Right then', he said to me. 'You've got five minutes.'

Outwardly I nodded, pulled the hat back from my eyes, said 'OK' and waddled towards Emma. Inwardly I thought 'Fuck'.

I looked down at her and we smiled at each other. 'OK', I said, 'you know what to do.' She looked into my eyes and as we both breathed deeply she closed her eyelids. I gently took her into trance and began to create hypno-anaesthesia. The surgery lights were shining down on her, the machinery in the room was whirring and beeping. She had already drunk the dye which would enable the surgeon to see what was happening in her body throughout the operation on a TV monitor screen on the wall. Of course, the dye had caused the problems in the previous two operations, and I could see that she looked a bit 'green around the gills' as sailors would say when describing seasickness. I was worried that if she started to vomit there was a possibility that she would come out of trance and everything would be ruined, and the anaesthetist would be triumphant. As she drifted into hypnosis though, her skin colour became more neutral, then paler, and then she had the standard reddening of the skin on her cheekbones, a classic sign that she was nicely in trance.

I continued to give her suggestions that her body would be completely relaxed throughout the procedure, that she would be aware of everything and would be able to respond to any requests of the medical team, but that she would focus more on my voice than anything else. Her body softened, her breathing slowed, and she began to relax deeply. I then began the process of disassociating her, which means to take her mind out of her body. In my planning for the day, I was intending to use a classic disassociation technique, which was to get her to imagine that she floated up out of her body, up to the ceiling and to move to a corner of the room. From there she could just observe calmly everything going on in the theatre down below. However, it suddenly struck me that to imagine watching the operation from on-high possibly wouldn't be a pleasant thing to do. I therefore asked Emma to nod her head when she felt that she had floated up out of her body, and when she did this I began to improvise further and asked her to imagine floating up *through* the ceiling, and then up through every floor of the hospital. As she was doing this I looked up at the surgeon and told him that Emma was ready. Talk about working fast – only five minutes and she was in trance, anaesthetised and disassociated. I was so pleased that we had rehearsed everything in advance; otherwise, five minutes would not have been enough.

Whilst the surgical team commenced with their procedures, I continued to suggest to Emma that she was floating up through all 13 floors of the hospital and out of the roof into the sky. I reckoned that if she could stay as far away as possible from the actual physical aspects of the surgery, she would be unaware of what was being done to her body and therefore less likely to react negatively to anything. I asked her to keep floating up through the sky above the city, and then to go higher and higher through the stratosphere and up into outer space.

Whilst this was happening, I was doing my best just to focus on Emma so that I could read her body language and make sure that she stayed calm and relaxed, and to be ready for any signs that things were going wrong in case I had to react to keep her in trance and anaesthetised. However, I was also interested in what was going on around me, and I happened to look round at the surgeon at exactly the same time that he took a scalpel and made a large slit into Emma's groin. As the flesh parted a stream of blood sprayed into the air like a geyser of crimson-coloured water, and I suddenly remembered that I don't like blood. And when I write that, I mean that I *really* don't like blood. It was not the best moment to have a life-long squeamishness about blood, veins and hospitals kick in. My body immediately went into shock and I turned green; then varying shades of purple, yellow and finally as white as a sheet. I began to sweat, and I felt sick and light-headed. I began to remember the time when I was 16 and visiting a friend in hospital who had been badly injured in a car accident. As I sat by his bedside I started to pass out and I slid slowly under his bed. The nurse who had to pull me out and bring me round was unimpressed and told me that she had enough problems with the patients without the visitors causing trouble too, thank you very much.

Desperately I tried to create saliva in my dried-out mouth and to breathe deeply, but I was fighting a losing battle. All I could think about was that I had to stay in control so I could keep Emma in trance; I was responsible for everything going well and if I suddenly fainted and slumped across her body on the operating table it would rather spoil things. Fortunately, as I started to sway backwards and forwards the surgeon happened to look up. 'Are you alright?' he said.

'Erm, not really' came the feeble response from my parched lips. 'Get him a stool' he commanded and quickly I was plonked down onto a stool which they placed next to the operating table. I breathed a sigh of relief and slowly started to come round. I decided not to look at what the surgeon was doing anymore and just concentrate on my job. I continued talking to Emma, asking her to imagine floating through space, her body free and light, and I took her on an imaginary journey around the universe, moving serenely past the planets and stars. I was able to regain my composure and she lay calmly on the table whilst the surgeon got on with his work.

I asked Emma's subconscious to allow the plastic tube that he was threading through her blood vessels to pass easily and directly up to the liver. I could see the workings of her body on the monitor and I asked her to imagine that it was like a road map, and all of the veins and arteries were like roads. I then asked her to imagine that one of the veins could become larger, like a motorway in the midst of all the minor roads, and this motorway ran directly up from the groin to the liver. This motorway could be the route that the plastic tube took to take the coils to the tumours, in order to starve them to death.

Everything was going well after my initial fit of the vapours. After around half-an-hour though, Emma started to swallow and her brow furrowed. 'I think I'm going to be sick', she whispered to me. She looked very uncomfortable, and her body became tense. The surgeon stopped what he was doing and looked at me. This was the last thing any of us wanted as it could wreck the entire procedure. I breathed deeply and quickly began to give her suggestions that her body would let go of any feelings of sickness and that she would go into an even deeper state of calmness. Emma looked confused for a few moments before her body softened again and she went deeper into trance. She breathed deeply; the surgeon breathed deeply, I breathed deeply, everyone in the room breathed deeply. Only the anaesthetist looked crestfallen; her big chance to step in and save the day was snatched from her grasp.

I continued talking quietly to Emma, keeping her out of her body as she journeyed around the universe and the surgeon threaded a plastic tube into her. That slight feeling of sickness was the only moment of crisis throughout the whole operation, which went like a dream. The plastic tube had gone relatively easily through her blood vessels and he was able to inject the coils successfully. The whole thing took only 90 minutes (whereas previously it had taken over two and a half hours each time) and Emma had not been sick once. At the end of the operation, as the anaesthetist sullenly stomped off with a scowl on her face, the surgeon turned to me and said that he was absolutely astonished at what he'd witnessed. He said that it had been like operating on a dead body as there had been no defensive reflex movements from Emma at any stage. I think we were both breathing big sighs of relief – him because his previous two attempts had been such disasters, and me because it had gone without a hitch (apart from me nearly causing a major emergency near the start!).

'Give me one of your business cards', he said, 'we need to talk about this.' I gave him my card but I'm still waiting for that call all these years later.

Emma recovered quickly after the surgery and was out of hospital two days later and she continued to get healthier and stronger. A few years later she was able to get pregnant and to give birth (using hypnosis) to a strapping baby boy.

Emma is the bravest woman I've ever met. She is now, as I write this, 26 years past her 'die-by' date.

Chapter 4

'Don't Look Him in the Eyes'

I didn't set out to become a Hypnotherapist. In fact, when I was coming to the end of my school days back in the mid-1970s the Careers Master quite omitted to mention it as a suitable vocation for a lad with a grammar school education, a ready wit and shoulder-length hair. In fact, I don't think the Careers Master mentioned the possibility of becoming a Hypnotherapist to any of my school pals either. That could have been because he wasn't really a specialist in advising on career paths to adolescents (he was the Religious Education teacher who was given the job because he didn't have as many lessons as the other teachers). He actually knew very little about possible career choices. My interview with him went something like this:

Teacher: 'Ah, Briggs, nice to see you.'

Me: 'It's Burgess, sir.'

T: 'Ah, yes, of course. Now, what do you want to do when you leave school next year?'

Me: 'Dunno, sir.'

T: 'OK, well is there anything that you're good at or anything that you like doing?'

Me: 'I like reading.'

T: 'Ah, good. You like books, eh? Then I think you should become a librarian.'

Me: 'Oh, right. Thank you sir.'

T: 'Fine, so that's all good. Send in the next boy on your way out will you Briggs.'

Me: 'It's Burgess, sir.'

T: 'Er, yes, of course.'

And that was it. Fortunately, I didn't take his advice.

The path to my long career as a Hypnotherapist was an unlikely one as I only fell into the job by accident. I was the director of a publishing company in the early 1990s which went bust and I had to do something quickly to earn money. My dad had stopped smoking by using hypnosis and as a scientist he couldn't make sense of how it had worked for him. He'd tried to stop smoking many times before with no success, but how was it that some bearded bloke (all the best Hypnotherapists sport beards by the way — including the women — it's part of the apparatus of the Hypnotherapist, along with staring eyes and a monotone voice) had got him to lay down in a chair, relaxed him by talking softly to him and he hadn't wanted a cigarette ever since? This didn't compute with his left-brain, analytical view of the world so he started to read about hypnosis. He became so fascinated with the subject that he eventually trained in it and began practising privately from home, working on friends and family.

Did I 'fancy having a go at it' he asked me one day when I was considering my options. 'Why not', I thought, it seemed better than working for a living. I then went on a couple of training courses and set up my own private practice in East Yorkshire. Thus began a strange odyssey which so far has lasted over 30 years and which has changed my life (and, I like to think, the lives of some of my clients too) beyond recognition.

My work has taken me into the far-flung corners of the mind and in my time, I've used hypnosis to help people do simple things like lose weight, overcome phobias and stop smoking, as well as more exciting and unusual things like breast enlargement, surgery without anaesthesia, helping with cancer and past life regression. I've hypnotised people who have been abducted by aliens, I've spent time in prison with murderers, and I've appeared many times in the press as well as on TV and radio. I've given therapy to fellow trekkers on the Great Wall of China and on the Inca Trail in Peru on the way to Machu Picchu. I've also presented a conference paper about past life regression to Native American health workers on the Navajo reservation in Arizona. It's certainly been an interesting job, quite different to what I expected all those years ago when I first started to see clients (and I hope you find reading about it interesting too!).

Yet the most important aspect of it all is that many people who have come to me for treatment have got better; sometimes when they've tried everything else and I have been their last resort. I always feel very moved when a client says 'thank you, you've changed my life'. And 'getting a result' for people still excites me every working day.

But there are down sides to a career in hypnotherapy. I have become sick and tired of people shouting out 'don't look him in the eyes' whenever they find out what I do for a living (as you can imagine, parties can be hell when I hear this for the hundredth time). I also feel uncomfortable with people who think that I can control them merely by looking at them, or that as a Hypnotherapist I can walk on water.

Of course, there is still a perception in the minds of many people that hypnosis is something paranormal or supernatural, and I'm sure some people believe that I can bring the dead back to life. Though having said that, I've never tried it. Maybe if I did…?

OK, we *can* heal the sick by using hypnotherapy, but we don't use the laying-on of hands (in which case we'd probably get sued) or have angelic choirs singing in the background during a therapy session. Hypnotherapy is not some form of New Age belief system, but a totally natural form of healing which uses the deep, inner mind to help people to get better. I'll explain more about it as we go through the following pages. It has a substantial body of scientific research to support its benefits.

Chapter 5

'Are You Going to Put Me Under?'

Having learned something of the power of hypnotherapy by reading about Emma at the start of the book, you may be asking 'so what *is* hypnosis? What is trance?' There are so many myths and misconceptions about hypnosis that it might be best to tell you what it is *not*.

Firstly, it is not a sleep state or a coma. It is different from being under anaesthetic. You are usually not under the control of the hypnotist. It is not something weird or supernatural. It is usually not the case that after you come out of hypnosis you forget everything that happened whilst you were in trance. It is not a state in which you don't know what is going on around you.

So, if that is what it is not, just what is it?

I usually define it to my clients by saying that it is a focussed state of relaxed inner awareness; this means that as we go into hypnosis, we begin to become more focussed and most people in trance enter a state of relaxation. The trance can be of different depths as we can be in a light, medium or deep trance throughout a hypnosis session. You can think of it as going down a set of stairs: at the top of the stairs, you are wide awake; at the bottom you are fast asleep. As you step down the first couple of steps you begin to move into a light trance (or a light state of relaxation), if you keep going down the stairs you enter a medium state, and if you keep moving down the stairs you enter a deep state of hypnosis. If you keep going down the stairs after that you simply fall asleep.

When we are in hypnosis, we are usually still aware of everything that is going on around us, but we feel distant from it; we can react to the outside world simply by opening our eyes. I often say to my clients, 'forget coma, think relaxation; that way we'll be on the right track'. Having said that, here is a definition of hypnosis from the American Psychological Association:

> Hypnosis is a procedure during which a health professional or researcher suggests that a client, patient, or subject experience changes in sensation, perception, thought, or behaviour. The hypnotic context is generally established by an induction procedure. Although there are many different hypnotic inductions, most include suggestions for relaxation, calmness, and wellbeing. Instructions to imagine or think about pleasant experiences are also commonly included in hypnotic inductions.
>
> People respond to hypnosis in different ways. Some describe their experiences as an altered state of consciousness. Others describe hypnosis as a normal state of focused attention, in which they feel very calm and relaxed. Regardless of how and to what degree they respond, most people describe the experience as very pleasant. Some people are very responsive to hypnotic suggestion and others are less responsive. A person's ability to experience hypnotic suggestion can be inhibited by fears and concerns arising from some common misconceptions. Contrary to some depictions of hypnosis in books, movies or on television, people who have been hypnotised do not lose control over their behaviour. They typically remain aware of who they are and where they are, and unless amnesia has been specifically suggested, they usually remember what transpired during hypnosis. Hypnosis makes it easier for people to experience suggestions, but it does not force them to have those experiences. (American Psychological Association, 1994).

I'm not sure if that helps, but it does give a flavour of what hypnosis is.

One of the most irritating things we often hear as Hypnotherapists when a client comes out of trance is 'was I under?' They always use that bloody word 'under'! I can spend 20 minutes explaining to a client before they go into trance most of what I've written above, and they still expect to be 'under' – which means to be under anaesthetic, to be in a coma or sleep state or under my control. I spend a lot of time emphasising that hypnosis is totally natural. We all go into hypnosis at least 24 times a day; when we daydream, for example. Or when we are focussing on the TV, or reading a book or watching a movie. If we go on 'automatic pilot' when we are driving, that too is trance. Meditation is a form of trance. Drifting into and out of sleep is trance. Doing a visualisation at the end of a yoga session is trance. All of these experiences are perfectly natural and are all trances; in not one of them are we 'under'!

Also, almost everyone can be hypnotised. The only people who can't be hypnotised are those who are drunk or stoned (they are already in an altered state of awareness) or mentally sub-normal. If you ever hear some smart-Alec telling you that their mind is too powerful and they cannot be hypnotised, they are talking nonsense. If someone says that a hypnotist tried to hypnotise them but they couldn't be hypnotised, it either means that the hypnotist was crap or (more likely) that they resisted the process because they were scared of letting go.

There are four 'abilities' that people have with regards to hypnosis. Some people are naturally very good at hypnosis. This means that they have a natural ability to go into trance, much in the same way that some people have a natural ability to play sport or to play a musical instrument. Around 25–30% of people are naturally hypnotisable, and I call these Number Ones.

Some people are good at going into hypnosis; not as quickly or as easily as Number Ones, but still relatively smoothly. These I call Number Twos. Most people are average at hypnosis, which means they can still go into trance, but they tend to take a bit longer to get there and are usually more conscious throughout the process (Number Threes). Only a few people are rubbish at hypnosis (Number Fours), and these tend to be people who are very resistant to letting go (usually, I'm sorry to say, these are often men who have control issues).

Most people really enjoy being hypnotised once they have got used to it. Often, they don't want to come back to full awareness at the end of a session. What often surprises people is how normal the whole process of being hypnotised is. What they expect is swinging watch chains and staring eyes; what they get instead is a nice feeling of peacefulness. Occasionally a client will come out of trance at the end of a successful hypnotherapy session and say 'I don't think I was under' (I have to restrain myself from hitting them with a hammer as they say *that* word), 'I could hear every word you said; I could have opened my eyes if I wanted.' 'Exactly', I reply through gritted teeth, 'I told you that trance is natural, that you would merely be relaxed but not in a sleep state.' Hypnosis is simply a way of tuning into our inner world, without letting go of our outer world.

By letting go in this way and going inside ourselves, tuning out the outside world and tuning into our inner world, we tap into the subconscious (also known as the unconscious) mind. You may be wondering what the difference is between the conscious and the subconscious minds. I usually explain by saying that the mind is like an iceberg – the tip of the iceberg above the waves is the conscious mind; the bulk of the iceberg below the waves is the subconscious mind. We access the subconscious in most cases by relaxing and going beneath the surface of the waves.

Our conscious, thinking mind is about .0001% of the mind; our subconscious is around 99.999% of the mind. This is why hypnosis is so powerful, because when we are in trance we are using the powerhouse of the mind, the engine room of the mind. Recent research suggests that the conscious mind takes on board 50 bits of information per second, whilst the subconscious takes on board 11 million bits of information per second!

Our conscious mind contains many memories, but it's said that our subconscious contains memories of everything we have ever done, and this is why hypnosis is such a great way to regress back into them. I believe that the subconscious also stores memories from our previous lives and our ancestor's lives too. It is also the seat of our imagination and our emotions, which is why when we are in hypnosis it is easier to access our emotional pain than it is when we are in a more conscious state.

In spite of the countless people who have gained real benefit through seeing a Hypnotherapist, or whose lives have been transformed as a result of hypnotherapy; in spite of the many scientific papers on how the brain works when someone is in trance and the benefits of hypnosis, there still exists in the minds of some people the misapprehension that hypnosis is something unnatural or belongs to the world of the paranormal ('don't look him in the eyes!'). It beggars belief that the BBC's guidelines to their producers places hypnotism in the same category as exorcism, the Occult and the paranormal!

Check out the following piece of drivel which was pushed through the letterbox of my office a long time ago:

DANGER – HYPNOSIS

Hypnotism is a highly popular and seemingly harmless remedy for many minor problems and ills. By some this practice is regarded as 'a bit of fun'.

The problem with all this is that we are not told the real or whole truth. We must be more informed about these things and to be warned of another side of them. This is not an attack on any individual, but upon a system which we as Christians believe is **POSITIVELY HARMFUL.**

Hypnotism is of demonic origin and through the complete elimination of will power and conscious use of the senses, hypnosis is a most effective way of opening the door to all sorts of evil spirits. This power to literally take over possession or control of someone else is a witchcraft or occult phenomenon. Such domination is a misuse of personality. As human beings we were made to exercise control or authority over ourselves through that invaluable commodity of human personality called the will. Personality is like a machine, if we use it in a way it was not designed for, a breakdown will result. Human beings are also damaged when misused; hypnosis misuses personality because it turns people into robots and opens the personality to evil infiltration.

The true nature of hypnotism is further indicated by the fact that many hypnotists are also involved in other occult practices, such as automatic writing, astral projection, pendulum and Ouija board.

The power behind hypnosis is not a natural one but a supernatural one. Such a power can only come from one of two sources. From God, who loves mankind, or from Satan and his demons who seek to frustrate and lead astray, in order that they may eventually destroy. Supernatural or psychic power must come from the supernatural beings and not from within natural beings as we are wrongly told.

The hypnotist can so subject the will of the person to his own that he may control his thinking and behaviour. People in hypnotic states become empty; hypnosis literally overrides all the senses of the body to a point where you could even make someone kill. The reason Parliament passed the 1952 Hypnosis Act which limited stage displays of hypnotism, was because two women needed extensive psychiatric treatment after such a session.

We would ask the reader to consider the one true LIVING GOD who has been revealed in the LORD JESUS CHRIST. Have you ever thought seriously about the fact that you can know Jesus and his power in a personal way?

It then concludes with a quotation from the Bible and the name and address of a local evangelical church.

Such ludicrous nonsense just goes to show that the world of hypnosis still has some way to go to overcome certain delusions in the eyes of some members of the public.

Anyway, that's a bit of information about what hypnosis is (and what it definitely is not). The 'therapy' part of the word 'hypnotherapy' is what we do to help someone to get better when they are in hypnosis, and there are many different approaches and techniques that a Hypnotherapist will use.

The simplest (and most basic) method is called 'post-hypnotic suggestion therapy'. In this, the aim is to re-programme the subconscious mind to change whatever negative behaviour a client has been doing into a more positive behaviour. This is used often for problems such as smoking cessation and nail-biting. It can and does work very well for most people, but the problem is that solely using suggestions to overcome a problem is not working on the causes of the problem. This can mean that even if the suggestions appear to work and the client (for example) stops biting their nails, there is a possibility that the subconscious anxiety or anger that caused the nail biting in the first place will return in the future so they will start biting their nails again. Or worse still, the client stops biting their nails but the negative emotion causing the problem will come out in another way, for example by causing depression or skin problems.

This is the main reason why I prefer to use regression to help many of my clients with their issues. Regression simply means to go back into the past (and is, of course, something we all do naturally when we remember the past), but in regression therapy we are usually going back in trance to release the emotions that are stored in the emotional pressure cooker in our mind.

Another form of therapy which many of us use are techniques that come under the label of NLP (which stands for the rather cumbersome title of Neuro-Linguistic Programming). These techniques often use the speed of the mind to create rapid change in a person. They can be very successful, but again they don't work on the emotional causes of a problem.

What often surprises many people are the wide range of issues that hypnotherapy can help with. Most people know that it can help people to stop smoking (often in just one hypnotherapy session) or to lose weight or let go of stress, and many people understand that it is a very effective way to treat anxieties and phobias, but did you know that it can also be a way to heal physical illnesses or reduce pain? That it is proven to significantly reduce Irritable Bowel Syndrome (IBS) and that regression therapy can heal depression?

This is a list of some of the problems that hypnotherapy can be useful with:

Anxieties and panic attacks
Phobias and fears
Skin problems
Physical illnesses (including migraines, asthma and cancer)
Lack of confidence and self-worth
Sexual problems
Alcohol addiction and substance abuse
Weight issues
Behavioural problems
Smoking addiction
Stress
Irritable Bowel Syndrome (IBS)

Relationship challenges
Pain
Breast Enlargement

Yes, you read that last line right! It isn't just there to catch your attention (although I know that it *did* catch your attention). Surprisingly enough, hypnosis is an effective way to increase the size of a female's breasts. Hardly anyone knows about this little-known use of hypnotherapy (even most Hypnotherapists know nothing about it) but I have helped a number of women to get bigger boobs by using the power of their minds. 'How can this be possible?' I can almost hear you thinking. My research into hypnosis for breast enhancement goes back to 1949, when it appears to have been used for the first time on 20 women. 17 out of the 20 showed an increase in size of up to one and a half inches (almost four centimetres). 17 of them had an increase of around two inches (five centimetres)! Another successful use of hypnosis was carried out in 1974, when 13 women averaged an increase of over two inches.

So how does it work? It's quite simple. The mind and body are completely inter-linked; the connections between one's mental and bodily processes are real and anatomical. Our thoughts, beliefs and attitudes can alter the levels of our hormones and neurotransmitters. Neurotransmitters are the chemical messengers that carry all communication between our cells and that largely govern the activity of many of our physical processes. Our thoughts, beliefs and especially our imagination are not just fleeting images, but are electrochemical events which affect your mind and body. If a woman, often enough, imagines changes taking place in her breasts, and is able to regularly imagine the feeling of her breasts receiving warmth, energy and nutrients, then over time what she is imagining in her mind starts to take place in her body. I usually find that with regular breast enhancement hypnosis sessions the breasts start to grow from between eight to twelve weeks after starting such a programme. Often, not only do the breasts become bigger and firmer, but the women also notice a reduction in their waist size too.

Anyway, if you're able to get the thoughts of women's breasts growing larger out of your mind, I'll now get on with the rest of the book. Hopefully the above explanation as to what hypnosis is and is not has been useful, so that what follows in the coming pages will make more sense.

Chapter 6
Hilary's Story

In order to demonstrate the ways in which hypnotherapy can help with psychological issues, let me share with you one of my case studies. I've often written about how incredible hypnotherapy is when it works really fast to help a client to overcome their problems. However, there are other cases where the Hypnotherapist needs stamina as it may take quite a lot of sessions before the client is healed. One such case was my client Hilary, who had a 'cluster' of problems, all of them caused by anxiety. She was claustrophobic, ground her jaw every night in her sleep, and she also suffered from trichotillomania.

She remembered that she had always had claustrophobia (the fear of enclosed spaces), even as a child. This phobia was especially strong if she had to get into a lift (elevator) or if she was in a crowd of people. She used to have panic attacks if she was in a crowd, and as well as this she hated having to wear tight things on her head, being physically restrained or anyone touching her throat. Her dentist was concerned for her teeth which were gradually being ground down in her sleep (she would wake up in a morning with her face aching and tight). Her form of trichotillomania was unusual too. This usually takes the form of an irresistible urge to pull hair out of one's head. However, in Hilary's case she was regularly pulling out her eyelashes.

The causes of these issues were a range of things: some significant emotional events from her childhood and adolescence (at an early age she had to become her mother's caregiver); some difficult and abusive relationships with men; a husband who caused her a great deal of stress because of his ability to make every challenge in his professional life a catastrophe. I used a variety of techniques to treat her, mainly using regression to release her locked-in anxieties and anger, but also EFT (about which more later) and some NLP too. Over time she became much calmer and more balanced, and the claustrophobia and urge to pull out her eyelashes died right down and she became free of them.

However, the teeth grinding remained and it was when we started to work in regression in past lives and her ancestors' lives that this was released. She relived several previous lives, all of which contained traumas that were affecting her in this life by creating anxiety inside her. During the day, by keeping busy she could ignore the anxiety; when she was asleep it would come out in the form of teeth grinding. In the first past life she was a young male who was waiting for his fiancée to arrive. When she didn't turn up, he felt very anxious; this turned to grief when he found out that she'd been killed in an accident involving horses. In the next life she was a man in 1960s America. The car showroom he was working in was engulfed by fire and he died in an explosion.

If this is your first introduction to the concept of Past Life Therapy then stay with me on this, as there is much more to come later on. Almost certainly by the end of this book you'll have a much deeper knowledge of what it is and how it works.

The third past life was significant in other ways. In this, she again was a male, and she was living in an industrial city in England in the 1800s. When she was in trance, I asked her to describe to me what she was experiencing:

It's daytime and I'm walking purposefully down a busy street with town houses on either side. I'm dressed smartly, with clean, black shoes. My clothes feel starchy and stiff and I have a hat on my head. I walk past some iron railings in front of a park and into an office. I think it's a legal office. I have plans or papers rolled up in a hardback book. I walk upstairs to an office and put the papers on a desk. I'm explaining things on the papers to a man; we're laughing and shaking hands. Once we've finished our business I leave there feeling light and successful. I have a busy mind; thinking about the next stage of whatever it is that I'm involved in. I go home to where I live with my younger sister — she's called Meg. There's a photo of our parents on the wall; they're dead and I feel sad but proud that I'm carrying on father's work. I feel close to my sister and we're talking about my success. My hands feel quite rough, as if I'm used to manual work. We design and plan things but we build them as well. We have an industrial building with machinery in it. I'm moving the family business up to a new level, into a bigger factory.

Hilary paused and was silent for a while as if she was moving on in time; then she went on:

It's night time and I'm sat in an office at a wooden desk and the walls are wood panels. I'm tired as I've been working hard. I'm looking at a sheet of paper with lots of numbers on it. A window looks into a big factory with lots of machines in it. I'm trying to figure something out. I feel heavier than before, stressed with business worries. My brow is wrinkled and I'm frowning. My chest feels tight and painful.

Again, Hilary was quiet for a time and she continued:

I've moved on in time. I'm older and I'm in the factory. There are big pistons going and lots of movement and noise and dirt. The machinery's black with grime and there's steam. My office looks down into a big, long building and there are skylights at the top letting light in. It's hot. There are other offices with men like draughtsmen and planners working in them and people working on the factory floor. I feel heavy and tired, stressed. I'm troubled and tense. I'm old before my time. I feel less stressed when I'm on the factory floor talking to the workmen.

Hilary paused, her face set and serious and her brow furrowed. She looked extremely uptight and uncomfortable. I could see her jaw clamped tightly together and mouth moving side to side, as if she were grinding her teeth. Her hands were tight fists in her lap. Soon she continued:

I've gone onto a later time now. I'm sitting in my office with my head in my hands, despondent. The factory is silent, all the machinery has stopped. It feels cold. I'm walking outside in the snow with a big overcoat and hat on. The business has gone bust. It feels like a final walking away, not looking back. I'm lying in bed now wearing a long white nightshirt. It's cold and there's a little lamp on a table next to the bed. I feel broken-hearted. I can't get out of bed and I feel aged by all of the stress. I have a stone-like feeling in my chest. I'm dying. I feel light now, and everything's bright. It's over.

Hilary breathed a sigh of relief and the tension that had been on her face throughout all of this eased away. She came out of trance saying she felt calmer than she had done for a long time. She said that she could now understand why she had so often felt depressed at certain periods of her life; the feeling of tension and hopelessness that she remembered from those times matched perfectly the feelings she'd felt in the past life.

Our next session worked on the next 'layer' of locked-in emotions causing the teeth grinding. In this session she regressed into the life of one of her ancestors. Her subconscious indicated that she had inherited trauma from a paternal great-

great-grandfather and once she was in trance she regressed back into his life. She relived this as if she was in his body, looking out through his eyes and feeling his feelings as if she were him:

It's daytime and I'm standing on the side of a dock looking at fishing boats. I feel around 30 years' old. I'm working; it's a busy place, people moving stuff on and off the boats. I'm wearing waterproof clothing, waiting for the tide so we can go out on a boat. I feel comfortable; this is my job and I know everybody here — the docks and working on ships feels like home. It's summertime and I'm excited as it's perfect weather for fishing. It's not my boat but I'm older than the rest of the crew; there are about six of us altogether. We'll be sailing from Hull, heading out on the Humber to the sea. We're holding big mugs of tea, smoking and laughing. It'll be a short trip, just a couple of days.

Hilary went quiet for a short time, as she moved on in time in his life. Speaking quietly, she continued with her narrative:

We're out at sea now, getting the nets and things ready to drop into the sea. Later on, we're putting fish into the hold, and then getting ready to come back into dock.

Once more she paused for a while before continuing:

It's another trip now, we're at sea and it's grey and wet. The boat's going up and down and there's water coming over the sides. I've got waterproofs on but they feel heavier than before. It's cold and wet but I feel OK.

Suddenly Hilary's face became serious and her body tense. Her head moved to one side as if she was trying to look behind her. Her words came faster than before and her breathing quickened:

> *One of the younger lads at the back of the boat is in trouble. Someone's gone to help him. I go to help out too. He's trapped or got some of his clothing stuck. We get him out of his waterproof but his jacket's stuck. Ah, a big wave's come and pushed him over the back of the boat into the sea. He's just in his shirt and trousers. I feel awful, shocked. We've got to turn the boat around to try to find him. The waves are really high; he appears and then disappears as we bob up and down. There's no knowing if he could swim. My chest feels tight. I feel responsible — if I'd been there earlier I could have grabbed him. It's slow turning the boat against the waves. We can't see him. I feel helpless. We're always aware of danger but I feel desolate, a deep sense of loss and the seriousness of it; I wish I'd been able to stop it happening. We're unable to find him, so we turn for home. Someone will have to tell his family. However, we're aware that it's a dangerous job and deaths do happen. He won't be the first or the last that it happens to. Even though I accept it we're all very quiet on the way back home. We arrive and empty the boat of the catch; we still have to get on with work regardless of the loss of life. The captain's heading off to tell the lad's parents. We're all quietly working and smoking; I feel subdued and thoughtful.*

Hilary sighed deeply as her great-great-grandfather's life slipped away out of her consciousness, and she slowly came out of trance and yawned. Afterwards she explained that she knew nothing of her father's family line, so she was unable to verify if what she had experienced was true, but she said that it felt so real that she was willing to accept it as a trauma that had come down to her in her genes. It was a trauma that her energy field could now let go of and allow her to heal.

When Hilary came for her next session, she was pleased to report that there had been some reduction in the intensity of her nocturnal teeth grinding, as well as her general anxiety. In this session, once she went into trance, her subconscious took her back into a past lifetime. Unlike many past life sessions, in which several major traumas are often uncovered and worked through (often the death in past lives is the cause of the problem that the client has in this present lifetime), we only got one single incident before the subconscious took her away from it. It was as if her inner mind knew that we had done enough to release the life.

I asked her to share with me the images that she was seeing in her mind's eye:

> *I'm outside looking at red skies, sand, scrub, bushes and round huts made from dried straw. It's very hot. I'm an adolescent girl, around 14 years' old, watching some children playing at sunset. It's tribal and I'm dark skinned; maybe Africa. There are people cooking on fires and I'm hungry. People are wearing traditional clothes as well as some modern clothes — it's not a village that's untouched by modern society. There's a cheerful, bustling energy. It's dark now, everyone sitting around fires, although there's some electric supply from generators* (obviously this was a relatively modern past life). *It's late at night now and it's very quiet. I'm lying inside a circular, one-roomed hut with my family. I can hear men's hushed voices outside, urgency in their voices. They're talking about something significant; guns or rifles or something.*

She was quiet for a while, and when she spoke she had moved on in time:

> *It's daylight, early morning and it's damp and cooler. The men have all gone and so has the jeep. The adults are all very anxious*

and quiet. The day gets hotter and brighter, with people trying to stay out of the sun. Kids are jumping into the river from some rocks to cool down; women are washing bowls and clothes in the river. Usually they're happy but this time they're all quiet and nervous. The men don't come back and it gets to night time and there's still no jeep. We sit round the fires and people are chatting a little but there's tension in their voices. I can feel a lot of anxiety in my chest and my jaw.

Throughout all of this Hilary had gradually become more and more tense. Her face was frowning and tight, her body was stiff and her breathing was rapid. Even though there didn't appear to be anything massively traumatic happening in the past life, the young girl in the African village was feeling extremely uptight.

I don't think what's happening is personal to me but I can feel everyone's stress. The night goes on and the lights are kept on; the women are staying up, waiting. There's a wariness, an edginess to the place. You could cut the tension with a knife and I can feel it in my body. Eventually we see lights on the road; a vehicle coming. The men are back, but not all of them.

Tears began to stream down Hilary's cheeks as she quietly cried. Her hands were clasping and unclasping as she felt all of the young girls' pain and agitation.

Two of them have been killed. Everyone is wailing and moaning. I'm crying, feeling very nervous and anxious. The whole village is in mourning, and everyone is frightened. Something has changed and something is going to happen. I don't know what's going on, but we're all very scared.

Again, she paused for a while whilst the tears flowed, and then she began to relax.

I don't know what's going to happen but the pictures have gone, it's as if I can't see anymore and I can't get it back.

This was her subconscious' way of saying that we had done all that we needed to do. Even though it felt incomplete, her subconscious mind didn't want her to go back into that past life in any of our other sessions (in fact in the next session it indicated that there was nothing else to do in that life as it was fully cleared) and she came out of trance. Hilary did feel very calm though, even if she was puzzled as to what else happened in that lifetime and we finished the session with a slight air of bewilderment.

Once more, when we met a few weeks later Hilary was pleased that her teeth grinding was reducing. On some nights it still happened but when she woke each morning her face and jaw were much less tight than they used to be. This time, once she went into hypnosis and relaxed, her subconscious took her into another ancestor's life; as before, it was three generations ago, an episode in the life of her maternal great-great-grandfather. As she started to share the experience with me, her speech was rapid and clipped and her body became tense:

There's a big, metal ship's door and I can't open it to go through. I'm pacing up and down feeling very frustrated. I'm quite young, about 30, and I don't know what to do. I'm hammering on the door and shouting; I can feel the anger in my throat. I've got a job to do because something has happened but I can't because the door's locked. Ah, finally it opens and I go in and along and then down narrow, metal steps. There are metal walls and it's a long descent down a steep staircase. It's very echoey. I can hear an engine, pistons going up and down. I go into a big engine room on board a ship. The noise is almost overwhelming. I'm wearing trousers and a shirt and a leather pinafore over the front to protect me. I have callused, worker's hands. The engine noise is constant. I have a feeling of immediacy, as if something has to be done and done quickly. I was frustrated earlier because I couldn't get started and I knew how urgent it is. I think it's last-minute repairs. I can see the arc light of welding going on. I'm waiting; I have to make sure that it's done. We're not at sea, the ship's being built and we're making sure the engines are working OK. I can feel the thudding and vibrating coming up through my body. We had to get the job done quickly, a major thing before the ship puts to sea.

Even though she was in hypnosis, throughout all of this Hilary was not relaxed at all, her body stiff and her face set. Although the scenes that she was experiencing were not unduly traumatic, her great-great-grandfather evidently felt a lot of anxiety as he raced against time to complete the work. Finally, though, she let out a big sigh.

We've finished and I breathe a sigh of relief. I was feeling so tense, it was a last-minute emergency job and I can relax now. It was very important to make sure the job was done properly; it had something to do with the structure of the ship. I go back up the metal staircase and outside on deck. I leave the ship with lots of workers. There are cranes, big ships and lots of metal everywhere. I smoke a cigarette as I walk out of the shipyard gate. I feel like a weight has been lifted off my shoulders.

Once more Hilary sighed, and as she came out of trance she yawned and stretched her jaw; it had felt so tense during the regression, she said. Once more, she knew nothing of her ancestor's life, but the tension and frustration had felt so real that she had no doubt that now that she had released it from her subconscious that she would feel much calmer in herself generally. With all of these past lives and ancestor's negative feelings inside her she could understand why she had such a tight jaw in her sleep. During the day she was busy and so therefore she didn't feel the tension inside her, but when she was asleep her subconscious tuned into it and her body reacted by grinding her teeth.

When Hilary returned for our next session she reported there had been further reduction in her teeth grinding, even waking up on some mornings with no tension in her face at all. She was happy that our therapy work was starting to show positive results. This time, when she lay in my reclining chair and I guided her into hypnosis, she went back into another past life. She shivered a little, as if feeling cold, as she spoke:

> *I'm in a village in the mountains, maybe in Scotland, a long time ago. It's a very poor place, about 20 small houses with rooves of mud and sticks. There's mud underfoot, no roads, and a river close by. There are horses and chickens moving around. I feel at home; I'm a young man, married but with no children. The weather's changing; winter's coming and we're getting ready for it. I'm stocking up with wood. My older relatives live in my house, partitioned off with curtains. Our coats are made from animal skins. We expect a hard winter as we've been reading the signs — the berries and the sky. All the men get together in a big hall — the place where animals are put in the winter to keep them safe — to discuss the things that need to be done. It's like a village council and everyone relies on each other, people work together.*

Hilary started to shiver more noticeably as she paused and moved on in time, and her voice hardened as she became more anxious:

> *The bad weather starts; it's really cold air. I'm on a horse with one or two others, heading away from the village to search*

for someone. We're looking to find my brother who should have come back. He was with a group that went hunting. We're in the woods, near a stream, shouting. I feel very anxious, wondering what's happened to him. There should be two horses as my brother was hunting with another man. Eventually we can see a fire with a man sitting next to it, but there's only one horse. I can feel a horrible pain in my chest, a feeling of loss and anguish. The man tells us that my brother's horse had an accident and he fell off and was injured and died. The man managed to pull his body from under the horse; the wolves came and ate the dead horse. The fire is keeping the wolves away from them. We walk back to the village with my brother's body on the horse. I feel terrible; pain and anguish. After we get back we have a funeral and then burn his body on a wooden rack; the ground is too hard to bury him. I can still feel the grief in my chest and a sense of loss. His death has devastated me. The snow is starting to fall now, the first snowflakes of winter.

Throughout most of this Hilary had tears running down her cheeks, but after a while she sighed and relaxed in the chair. The past life was over and she had released the painful emotions that she had bottled up inside her all of her life.

As I mentioned earlier, none of Hilary's past life and ancestral life experiences were, outwardly, very traumatic. In regression therapy my clients often get much bigger and unpleasant traumas coming through that can sometimes cause them to cry, to scream, to shake and occasionally even to writhe around whilst they are in trance re-experiencing the traumas. However, the overall anxiety and tension that was inside Hilary from the past was causing such locked-in emotions and up-tightness that she was subconsciously responding to it by doing her negative behaviours of eyelash pulling and teeth grinding.

As a result of our sessions, regressing into significant emotional events from this life, past lives and her ancestors' lives, Hilary was able to let go of her eyelash pulling and her teeth grinding. She not only stopped these behaviours, but she also felt calmer and much stronger in her everyday life.

Chapter 7
Iris' Story

In order to demonstrate how regression therapy can help to overcome physical illness, this is one of my most dramatic examples.

Iris was a 60-something year old woman who came to me suffering from cancer of the lip. She had heard me talk about the emotional causes of illness and she wanted to discover the traumas from her past which had caused her cancer. She was an advocate of natural therapies and she didn't want to go down the traditional medical route. I stand firmly in the Louise Hay (*You Can Heal Your Life*) camp when it comes to saying that illness has emotional causes, and whenever I work with any physical illness, I aim to help my client to release the negative emotions that their subconscious mind is holding on to. If this can be done, their energy field releases the locked-in energies from the past and then the healing process in the body can begin. It appears that we can hold these negative emotions in specific parts of our energy field, but sometimes the way the negative emotions come out is in a symbolic way. An example of the former, in which emotions are held in a particular part of the body, is my client, Toni, who had been experiencing lower back problems. Her case is written about in detail in my book *The Power of Past Life Regression*. She was in pain all the time but nothing had been able to help her (including massage, physiotherapy, chiropractic, acupuncture etc.) and she had even had surgery but the surgeon could find nothing at all wrong in her back that needed repairing. She came to me for help and in regression her subconscious took her into a past life in which she was a (male) Nazi soldier in WWII who was shot in the back by a Russian sniper and killed. Once she had re-experienced the death a few times her energy field released the trauma that had been brought through into this present life and the back problem was completely healed.

However, Iris' cancer of the lip was of the symbolic kind of illness. This means that there was no physical trauma from the past that had left its imprint upon her mouth or her lip, but that there was a symbolic meaning to her cancer. As we discussed this possibility, Iris was acutely aware of how this related to her upbringing in this life. Her sister had always been aggressive towards her and Iris had never fought back; she had (metaphorically speaking) 'bitten her lip' in order to keep peace within the family. She had always avoided conflict as a child at home and she felt that she had never been heard by her parents, who had often 'squashed' her in order to control her. This meant that she had blocked her natural instincts to speak or even shout out and all of that locked-in energy was now causing a blockage around her mouth and therefore causing the cancer.

A controversial book written about the symbolic aspects of illness is *The Healing Power of Illness* by Dethlefsen and Dahlke. They write that, in their opinion, cancer is caused by unexpressed (or suppressed) love; that is someone who cannot love themselves or others enough. In their view cancer is the symptom of misunderstood love. They say that the heart is the only organ in the body that is very rarely attacked by cancer; the symbol of love is? The heart!

Once we had spoken about this, Iris now had some new insights about the nature of the illness and how it connected to this life, which she could contemplate at a later stage after our session. A part of me wondered if we needed to regress into some of her childhood memories but once she went into trance her subconscious indicated that there were two previous lives that were connected to causing the cancer. Unusually, both of these fell into the symbolic aspects of the cancer too, although there were some negative emotions that needed to be released as well.

As she began to drift deeper into trance, she went quite quickly into the first of the past lives, and as she did so she lost all of the relaxation in her body that so far, she had been experiencing. She stiffened and her face looked stern and set. Her head moved slightly from side to side as if she were trying to remove something that was on her face. I asked her to tell me what she was experiencing. She spoke in rapid, staccato tones, her breathing fast and her jaw tight:

There's a man behind me, holding my mouth so I can't scream. I feel really scared and I'm trying to fight him off. I can't shout.

Her head and shoulders continued to move from side to side as if she were trying to get away from her assailant. I asked her to tell me about herself and where she was. In clipped tones she continued:

I'm a girl, around 18 years' old. I'm wearing a blue silk dress and I have blonde hair which is a wig. I'm in a stone building. I'm in shock. The man is a black man and he's strong. I think he's a servant. He lets me go and I walk away. I don't know what to do but I don't tell anyone. I'm above him. He wanted to kiss me but I fought him off. He's misread the signals; this is something to do with communication. At first, I keep it a secret but then I tell someone and they take him. He's on his knees and they kill him.

Iris' hands were twisted and knotted together, she looked as if she was going to cry but she held it in. Her body was tense as she said:

I feel so guilty. I feel sad. It's my fault.

She continued to be in this anxious state for a few minutes before she started to relax again. After a short time, she spoke once more:

> *I've moved into another life. I'm a beautiful black woman and I get raped when I'm on my way to the river to get water. There's a man behind the bushes waiting for me. I'm alone and he pulls me into the red mud. It's slippery and I'm fighting, trying to get away. He holds me down.*

Once more she was silent as she relived the rape. Her whole body was tense and she had a look of disgust on her face. Soon she continued:

> *He belongs to my tribe but when I go back I can't tell anyone otherwise no-one will want to marry me. I have to keep the rape a secret. Eventually I marry and have children and have a happy life.*

Iris started to relax again as the past life slipped out of her mind. We did some further work on healing both of those lives, especially letting go of the sense of hopelessness that she had felt in them. She also sent some healing energy to the young woman in the first past life, allowing her to forgive herself for causing the death of the man who had been killed because of her speaking out.

She let go of both of the lives as they were now cleared of their negative energies, and I asked her to consider the ways in which those lives connected to the cancer in this present life. The theme in both of them was about the trauma of speaking out. In the first life she had spoken out and someone had been killed because of it; in the second life she was unable to speak out because if she had her life would have been damaged. Now she could understand how her body in her present life had held onto that energy which had naturally been held (at a subconscious level) around her mouth, causing the lip cancer.

I brought Iris out of trance and we finished the session. She told me that she felt a lot clearer about things now and she knew that she had a lot of processing to do. She could see why she had remained silent as a child — *'If I speak my truth I will lose people and bad things will happen.'* She was planning on using kinesiology to continue her healing work, and I felt that this would help her a lot.

Several months later I received an excited message from Iris. She had been to the hospital to see her specialist:

> *Hi Steve, they cannot find the cancer anymore. During the summer it has disappeared. The deep, deep traumas I worked through with you were released.*

Iris had also used kinesiology and natural foods after I saw her, and she had spent more time walking in nature. She was now well again, and the cancer was no more.

Chapter 8

The Itchy and Scratchy Session (or How I Fail to Help Donald Pleasance)

Bill's wife, Rita, phoned me in some distress. I could hear the desperation in her voice. 'My husband has got a phobia of fleas', she said. 'And it's driving me mad. He's obsessed with fleas and it dominates our life. We can't go anywhere or do anything in case he sees someone carrying fleas on them. He's in his early 60s and he can't go to work anymore because of it. He just sits at home all day watching out for fleas. It's like a madness. I don't think that I can take much more of it, it's ruining my life and I've told him that if he doesn't stop I'm going to divorce him.'

'That sounds horrible', I said sympathetically, 'you must be having a terrible time. However', (and at this point I spoke confidently, hoping to reassure her) 'I've treated many different phobias over the years, usually very successfully. So, there's a good chance I can help your husband.' Rita sounded grateful for the hope I had given her and she made an appointment for Bill to come and see me.

Rita brought him and she sat in my waiting room whilst we had the session. Bill was a mild-mannered, shy man, balding and wearing a 1970s jumper and a 1950s tie. He sat opposite me looking very intently at me, as if he was trying to read my thoughts. Then he looked down and started slowly looking around the room, as if scanning the floor for something. He reminded me of the actor, Donald Pleasance, in *The Great Escape*; I wondered if he would tell me that he could see perfectly and he could see a pin on the floor near the wall. However, once he had completed the scan of the floor, he looked at me with a vacant, bemused expression on his face. He didn't speak, just sat staring at me expectantly.

I began by welcoming him and then I asked him to tell me more about his phobia of fleas. 'Oh', he said quietly, 'but I haven't got a phobia of fleas.'

Taken aback by this I said, 'but your wife said you have a phobia of fleas and that it was ruining your life.'

'No', he said softly, his voice a dull monotone and his gaze unwavering into my eyes as he started to remind me of Donald Pleasance as Dr Crippen. I could feel my flesh creep a little. 'No, I haven't got a phobia of fleas. I HAVE fleas.' He stopped and continued staring at me. I could have sworn that his eyelids hadn't blinked once since he sat in the chair.

Puzzled, I repeated 'you HAVE fleas?'

'Yes', he said, 'and they're not just on me but all around me. Our house is infested with them. And wherever I go I take fleas with me and pass them on to other people.'

'But your wife didn't say anything about this', I said.

'No', he replied, 'she says that there are no fleas in our house and that it's all in my mind. But I know they are there; I can see them.'

As he was silent again, I started to feel uncomfortable because I sensed I was in the presence of someone who was perhaps not of sound mind. He cocked his head to one side and stared at me again. This time he started to look like Donald Pleasance in *You Only Live Twice*. All he needed was a scar on his face and a white cat in his lap and he would be a dead ringer for Blofeld. Was it just me or did he have a more menacing look in his eye this time. Was it just me or did I hear the purr of a cat somewhere in the room? Was it just me or have I been watching too many Donald Pleasance movies?

I wasn't sure what to do next. Playing for time so I could gather my thoughts I asked, 'so you're not frightened of fleas?'

Once more the unblinking gaze and the slow monotone voice came back at me. 'No, I'm not frightened of fleas. I HAVE fleas.' After a long pause I asked if it would be OK if I had a quick chat with Rita. He nodded and smiled wanly. I left the room and talked to Rita who was sitting in my waiting room; I told her what Bill had told me. 'Oh yes', she said quickly, 'he's obsessed with fleas. He says that they're in our house, in our bed, everywhere. But they're not. There are no fleas anywhere. We don't even have a dog or a cat. The house is scrupulously clean and I once even had pest control services in to clean the whole house from top to bottom to try and convince him that there were no fleas, but he still believes that they are there. I don't know what to do anymore; I'm at the end of my tether. He just sits in his chair all day long thinking about fleas. It's like I don't have a husband anymore, just this madness.' As she spoke she was struggling to hold back the tears.

'Hmm', I said in a tone which hopefully suggested intelligence and professionalism, but which was probably undermined by the look of confusion on my face. I wanted to reassure her, but I was at a loss as to what to say. What could I do to help a man who was clearly delusional? I left Rita and went back into my office to Bill. He hadn't moved, he was just sitting in his strange, unblinking way with an air of weirdness around him.

'OK Bill', I said, trying not to sound challenging or patronising. 'Rita says that there are definitely no fleas in your house and that it's all in your head.'

'Yes, I know she does. But she's wrong. There are fleas in the carpets, the house is infested.' Again, the dead-pan expression and the unblinking stare as he closely watched my reaction. I wondered where I could go with this. I'm a Hypnotherapist, used to treating normal people with normal problems, not a psychologist working in a psychiatric institution. I tried to reason with him — 'But how do you know there are fleas and that you pass them on to other people?'

'Because whenever I'm talking to people, I see them scratch themselves after a while. And then I know that I've passed some of my fleas onto them.'

He was watching me even more intently as he said this. I realised that he was watching me to see if I scratched myself, which would confirm that he had passed some of his fleas onto me. 'Don't scratch yourself', I thought to myself, 'whatever you do, don't scratch.'

I remembered a friend of mine told me how he used to sell Kirby vacuum cleaners. These were very expensive vacuum cleaners that were sold by hard-sell commission-only salesmen who came to your home to demonstrate how powerful the cleaners were. He told me that he would first of all vacuum the downstairs of your home and then show you how much gunk it had picked up. If that didn't convince you to buy, he would take you upstairs to your bedroom and strip off your bedsheets. He would proceed to hoover your mattress.

Triumphantly, he would then open the canister and show you how much gunk he had sucked up from your mattress. As he was doing this, he would launch into a graphic description of bed bugs and how everyone has thousands of them living on their mattress. At the juiciest and most unpleasant part of his talk he would whip out from under his jacket a photo of a bed bug magnified 10,000 times. As he held the photo up of a bed bug the same size as a small mammal with its scaly body, enormous legs and scary antennae, he would scratch himself. That was a stroke (or a scratch) of genius! He said that in nearly every case as he scratched himself, the customer did too. And as they scratched themselves, he popped the closing sales question. And more people bought the machine at that point in his presentation than at any other time. Sneaky, but brilliant. There's something universally suggestive about an itch. In fact, I wonder if a part of you right now is subconsciously trying not to scratch yourself? You've heard of scratch 'n sniff books? This book could be the world's first itch and scratch book!

So, as I sat with Bill looking at me, scrutinising my every move, and gave myself the order not to scratch myself, I realised that it was not the best of suggestions. As soon as I thought this, an itch appeared on my back. 'Don't scratch it Burgess, or he'll know that what he's saying is true.' Then another itch started on my leg; then another on my right testicle (though I suppose there's nothing unusual in that. Most men seem to spend half of their adult lives scratching their testicles). I started to feel very tense. The itches around my body intensified and multiplied – on my face, on my left arm, on my backside. 'Don't scratch Burgess.' I tried to get rid of the one on my face by screwing up my cheek. It didn't work and now I looked as if I was gurning at him. I narrowed my eyes in a futile effort to deal with the itch on my forehead and I realised it looked as if I was developing a nervous tic. I tried to remain calm and reason with him but all the time a thousand itches around my body were screaming out to be scratched. With my hands clasped tightly into fists and my buttocks clenched tightly together I was struggling not to explode into a paroxysm of scratching. It was like being tortured. In the midst of my agony, I had a flash of inspiration:

'So, Bill, if you've got fleas then you must be getting bites all of the time. Can you show me your flea bites?'

'Aha, got you there' I thought as my left eye started to twitch, sweat appeared on my forehead and I held tightly onto the arms of the chair.

'Oh well', came the reply, delivered in a monotone voice that was becoming more annoying by the minute as every nerve in my body was screaming 'scratch me, scratch me you bastard'.

'I'm immune to them now as I've had so many. I must get bitten but they don't show on my body anymore.'

'But what about your wife and family? Don't they complain of having bites on them?'

He thought long and hard about that one, before finally telling me 'maybe they're immune too now. I see them scratching though so I know that the fleas are on them'.

I started to realise that this was a battle I was not going to win. Bill was clearly suffering from a delusional disorder. I asked him if he would like to have some hypnosis which might help him to feel more relaxed but he refused. He told me that as there was nothing wrong with him, why should he need to have hypnosis? By this stage I had had enough. I was aching to scratch every part of my body and to rub my back up against the door frame (in my mind I started to hear Baloo the bear from 'The Jungle Book' singing the 'bare necessities of life' as he rubbed himself up against a tree trunk). There was nothing I could do to help him. He refused to acknowledge that he had a problem and he was not going to let me do any work with him anyway. Also, I am not trained to treat such a psychiatric illness.

I took him out to Rita and told them gently that I couldn't help. Rita was obviously very disappointed but as I explained the situation she understood. I told her that I thought that they should get an Environmental Health Officer into their home to search for fleas. If such an expert couldn't find any then maybe Bill would be forced to question his delusional beliefs. Maybe also she could get a CBT therapist to work with him. It was the best I could do under the circumstances, and as they left my office (she sadly, he victoriously) I breathed a sigh of relief and spent the next 10 minutes vigorously scratching myself like a rabid animal.

I realise that I have written about this in a light-hearted way, but of course it was sad to see Bill unable to live his life without his mind being dominated by such a strange fantasy and obviously I was disappointed that I was unable to help him.

I share this peculiar episode in my professional life to show that all therapists have failures, and also to highlight that strange things can occur when you're working with human beings, with all of their foibles and idiosyncrasies.

Now, if you don't mind, I have to go and scratch myself all over.

Chapter 9

Warning: The First Sentence Will Grab Your Attention

One of the strangest periods of my career was in the early 1990s, when I spent three years in HMP Hull teaching meditation and stress management techniques to the inmates. In those days it was a Category 'A' prison, which means that it was a high-security prison, housing male prisoners who posed the highest threat to the public, the police or national security.

As you can imagine, I met some interesting characters in there, as well as some dangerous ones. I had some unusual experiences too. One of which included sitting cross-legged and with my eyes closed, meditating in the prison cell of a double murderer. Another was talking in solitary confinement to a former Hell's Angel convicted of paedophilia (an unpleasant, creepy experience).

Being in the prison system for so long changed my views of prisons and prisoners. Before I stepped into Hull prison, I naively thought that prisons were places in which inmates had an easy life and that they all deserved to be punished harshly for their misdemeanours. Now I know that prisons are very unpleasant places filled with people who often need healing and not punishment. Yes, I realise that there are some very dangerous people who have been locked up for serious crimes, many of whom show no remorse, and of course such criminals need to be held in prison to protect the public. However, time after time I met prisoners who were desperate for psychological help and some assistance that would give them a chance to adapt to a more functional life back in society upon their release. I read somewhere that a psychologist had interviewed thousands of prison inmates and found that 85% of them came from broken homes and abusive childhoods. She actually stated that she believed that the true figure should be higher than 85% but many of those she interviewed didn't want to admit or didn't understand that their childhoods had been dysfunctional. What this means to me is that, along with the social factors that drive young people into crime, the psychological factors should be addressed if we truly want to do something as a society to reduce crime.

In my opinion, many prisoners need to have therapy to heal their childhood wounds. They are often simply responding to their inner emotional pain by being anti-social. If their Inner Child is hurt and angry as a result of childhood abuse, then they react throughout their lives to that abuse by feeling angry and hurt. This is how we all behave as human beings, subconsciously responding to our childhood wounding.

And as for the idea that they have a chance of receiving rehabilitation whilst they are in the prison system, that really is just a myth put around by politicians to pretend that the government is doing something to reduce the prison population. In my opinion there is simply not enough money or motivation put into rehabilitation, and I don't think that there is any political will to change things. So, the cycle of crime and punishment just goes on and on.

Anyway, let me come to the real point of this section of the book by telling you about the time that I spent with Charlie Bronson, who is often called 'Britain's Most Violent Prisoner' by the tabloid press, which loves to write about him.

Charlie is now 71 years old and has spent more than half of his adult life behind bars (50 years so far). He was an armed robber, who after he was imprisoned staged roof-top protests in jails causing hundreds of thousands of pounds worth of damage. An incredibly strong man (I believe he does two thousand press-ups a day), he has spent months in cages in solitary confinement as well as having his sentence increased to life imprisonment for his activities (which includes hostage taking) both inside and outside prison. I have to say that despite his fearsome reputation, I got on very well with Charlie and I developed a high regard for him based on our time together. I admire his courage in overcoming often appalling conditions which he has faced over the years. Despite everything the prison system has thrown at him he hasn't cracked and they couldn't break his spirit. Tom Hardy made a creditable stab at portraying him in the 2008 movie *Bronson*.

I was part of a small team of teachers who worked with Charlie for four months whilst he was in 'A' Wing at Hull prison, and we found something in him that no-one had found before – that he is incredibly creative and a brilliant artist with an unusual style and an artistic vision which is unique. Nowadays, he calls himself Charles Salvador; a tribute to the great painter Dali. As Charlie and I got to know each other talking and playing chess he found out that I had been a freelance writer and also the editor of a business magazine; this prompted him to come up with the idea of us writing a radio play together.

And so we did – the concept was Charlie's and we corroborated on the script. Not surprisingly it was set in a prison and the main character was a man (we called him 'Charlie') who found himself sent down for a crime of which he has no memory. He believes himself innocent but soon after he is put into a cell, he begins to hear a voice (Charlie called this the 'Ego-voice') in his head. The Voice insinuates itself into his thoughts and begins to control him, at the same time gradually opening up the memory of the murder which he did actually commit. As we wrote it together Charlie played the role of 'The Voice' and I can still hear the chilling, wicked relish of his gravelly, cockney-like accent when I re-read the words of the play. Here's a small part of the script.

The character, Charlie, has been sentenced and in his first hours in a cell at the courthouse has attacked the officers after hearing

The Voice. He has been put in a strait jacket and left to await the secure van which will take him to Parkhurst prison. Lying alone and frightened he begins to talk to himself, all the time whimpering, sighing, sniffing etc.:

Charlie: Why me? I can't believe this. I can't move – what is this contraption? I can't move me arms; I'm all trussed up. They're treating me like a madman – I'm not mad. A strait jacket. Why are they doing this to me? I can't even pick me nose. (WHIMPERS) Life sentence. I can't breathe. (SHOUTS) I wanna go to the loo. (TO HIMSELF) I feel all dizzy, my eyesight's all blurring. Me mouth's all dry. (SHOUTS) Somebody help me. Where are you? Somebody get me out of here. Help; help!

Ego-voice: (MAD LAUGHTER)

Charlie: (SCREAMS) No, not you again.

Ego-voice: Come on Charlie, cool down. Just look at the state of you. You'll never survive a life sentence behaving like this.

Charlie: Who are you? Where are you?

Ego-voice: You know who I am and I'm here to stay; we're in this together.

Charlie: We? Who's we? There's no-one else here. You don't exist. You can't exist.

Ego-voice: Charlie boy, listen, and listen good.

Charlie: (WHIMPERS)

Ego-voice: What I'm about to tell you, you must come to terms with, 'cos if you don't you're never gonna see daylight again.

Charlie: (MOANS)

Ego-voice: You know Charlie, what you done.

Charlie: But I never done anything.

Ego-voice: Look at it this way, I was there, I saw you do it.

Charlie: Do what? I never did nothing.

Ego-voice: For God's sake Charlie, you put five bullets in his nut.

Charlie: Whose nut? What are you talking about?

Ego-voice: Look, it's now, I can help you. Do you want help? (PAUSE) Well, do you? (LOUDLY AND AGGRESSIVELY)

Charlie: (CONFUSED) Yes — no — I don't know. What do you mean?

Ego-voice: Well do you or don't you? Because if you don't, then you're on your own Charlie boy. And believe me, you ain't gonna make it on your own.

Charlie: No, please — help me — I want help.

Ego-voice: Right. Here's where we make a bond. I'll help you Charlie, on one condition.

Charlie: Condition? What's that?

Ego-voice: I'll get you out of that strait jacket and moved to a proper cell. They're treating you like a madman Charlie; you're in a padded cell. Now do you want me to get you out?

Charlie: Course I do, course I do; help me. HELP ME.

Ego-voice: I'll help you Charlie, but you're gonna owe me.

Charlie: Anything, anything, just get me out.

Ego-voice: Right, it's a deal. First, I'll tell you what you must do: once you're out of this padded cell, you must get a razor blade.

Charlie: Razor blade? What for?

Ego-voice: I'll tell you what for — you're gonna cut off one of your ears.

Charlie: WHAT?

Ego-voice: One of your ears Charlie, and you're gonna send it to the judge who sentenced you to life.

Charlie: One of my ears? I can't do that.

Ego-voice: You can do it, and you will do it.

Charlie: God, are you mad? You can't be serious.

Ego-voice: That's the deal – you agreed Charlie. Remember, there is no alternative, only this empty padded room, more injections, more hidings, more loneliness. God, look at you Charlie, you can't even wipe your own arse. It'll kill you, Charlie. (SHOUTS) It'll kill you. (PAUSE) Now, do you agree?

Charlie: Yes, don't leave me here – I wanna get out. Anything. (DESPERATELY) Anything.

Ego-voice: OK Charlie, say after me. I will…

Charlie: I will…

Ego-voice: Solemnly swear…

Charlie: Solemnly swear…

Ego-voice: To obey my master, my friend, my friendly master…

Charlie: To obey my master, my friend, my friendly master… (GETTING WILDER THROUGHOUT) My redeemer, my saviour.

Ego-voice: My redeemer, my saviour.

Charlie: My redeemer, my saviour. Anything, just get me out of here.

Ego-voice: Right Charlie boy, that's the deal done. I'm gonna get you out of here now. Listen, we ain't got much time; the doctor will be coming soon to see you and all those nasty men in white coats. Now you've got to play it cool; this is a big game Charlie – 'yes sir', 'no sir', 'three bags full sir'. You understand that?

Charlie: Yes, I think so.

Ego-voice: You play games with 'em, let 'em see that you can be manipulated. Let them see that you're willing to try. Let them know only what you want them to know. Tell 'em nothing and at the same time everything they want to hear.

Charlie: I don't think I can do it; I'm frightened. I need help, will you help me do it … will you help me?

Ego-voice: I'll help you. I'm your friend, remember? (SOUNDS OF KEYS RATTLING IN THE LOCK) Here they come Charlie, here they come.

I think that you have to agree that it's a pretty good piece of playwriting coming from a man who is popularly portrayed as an out-and-out villain. The play continues with the unfortunate Charlie settling into prison life with the ever-haunting Voice playing a more and more influential role in persuading him to take actions that become more and more catastrophic. Unfortunately, we didn't finish writing it because he took the deputy prison governor hostage (who I was told later had the habit of winding Charlie up whenever they talked). After an incident that lasted for 48 hours before the deputy governor was released, Charlie was taken to another prison and I didn't see him again. He then spent a long period being 'ghosted' from prison to prison within a short time in order to de-stabilise him.

As I was working with him on the play, Paul, one of Hull prison's art teachers, was working with Charlie too and his now-famous career as an artist began. It has been claimed by others that they were responsible for this after he left Hull, but the fact is that his time in Hull prison was the real catalyst for this. With Paul's help, Charlie wrote a book about various characters that he had met in prison over the years, which was printed and ring-bound in the art department.

Although Charlie has an awesome reputation as a hard man and of being violent and unpredictable, I always felt safe with him (we spent many hours alone together) and I relished his sharp sense of humour and his wry view of the world. One of my favourite stories told to me by Charlie about his life in jail (he calls prison a 'concrete coffin' as he wonders if he'll eventually die behind bars) is that of 'The Sweet Man'. Apparently, he was in the intensive care unit in a top security hospital and one of the inmates stood out for Charlie because he had a cold, hard stare and was always on the alert. Every day the man would go around the unit and offer the prison officers a boiled sweet from a bag of sweets that he kept with him. But he never offered a sweet to any of the inmates. This went on for months, with Charlie watching his behaviour day after day, becoming more and more irritated by the fact that the man only offered sweets to the warders. Eventually, Charlie had had enough and one day, when no-one was around, he grabbed the man and pinned him up against the wall. Angrily, he demanded why he never offered his sweets to Charlie and the other inmates. Terrified, the man stammered 'but I don't like the wardens, and I like you Charlie'.

Puzzled, Charlie released his grip on the man and asked, 'but if you don't like them, why give them sweets?'

'That's simple', he said. 'Each week I buy boiled sweets and each night in my cell I stick some up my arse and then wrap them back up again before giving them to the wardens the next day.'

Charlie let go of him and thanked him profusely for his good work.

Isn't that brilliant? I still remember tears rolling down my cheeks as Charlie acted out the tale to me.

At the end of our sessions together Charlie would insist on giving me a 'bruvver hug' and I would find myself hugging a man who is built like a bear and who could have crushed me like a grape, but I never felt threatened and I trusted him totally. Although we swapped letters for a couple of years after he was transferred from Hull, life took over for me and the letters stopped. A few years later I was in a bookshop and I happened to see Charlie's name on the spine on one of the books on the shelves. I took it down to find that he'd written his autobiography. As I flicked through the pages I wondered if he'd written about his time at HMP Hull. Imagine my surprise as I found that I was actually mentioned as he wrote about his experiences on 'A' Wing. I was incredibly moved as I read that he had a lot of respect for me and that I have a big heart. Thank you, Charlie, I am honoured by your words.

I count myself privileged to have met Charlie and to have shared his company and I sincerely believe that he should be released from jail; there are far worse individuals in the prison system who have committed far worse crimes and who have served much less time than Charlie and who have been released. He has never killed anyone, but he has developed a reputation for brutality which I feel is nowadays undeserved. As he moves towards the later stages of his life he appears to have changed and become much more contemplative than before. The Charles Salvador Art Foundation was founded to promote his artwork and 'help those in positions even less fortunate than his own' to participate in art, surely not the activity of someone who is simply a mindless brute. The compassionate thing that should be done, in order to show that we live in a humane society, is to set him free. As Charlie himself says, 'I've had more porridge than The Three Bears'. I can only hope that at some time soon his porridge days will be over.

Chapter 10

The Real X Files

In 2005 I was contacted by a researcher from a TV production company who had heard about my experiences as a regression therapist. They were producing a documentary for Sky TV which was to be called *The Real 4400*. This was about several people who claimed that they had had 'missing time' experiences as a result of alien contact or abduction. They asked me to regress a lady who felt that, together with her family, she had been abducted but none of them had any memories of it, other than seeing a space craft just before the experience happened. It sounded unusual so I agreed to be filmed doing the regression (the programme is still available on YouTube if you're interested).

As a result of giving some talks about regression to a local UFO Society, I had already met several people who claimed to have either seen alien space craft or even had contact with extraterrestrials. One of them, Andy McCartney, had some half-memories about something weird that happened one night as he left a pub in Hull (he was adamant that he was not drunk as he'd only had a couple of small bottles of beer). He had vague memories of being drawn into a sort of marquee and fighting off some beings in there; he also had a feeling that something had happened, but he didn't know what. He just knew that he felt a strange sense of unease whenever he thought about it. By the way, Andy is happy for me to use his real name as his case has already been featured in other publications.

He came to my office and he told me in more depth the few parts of the incident that he could remember. It took place on 26 December (Boxing Day in the UK) 1980. This proved to be a very significant date, but more about that later. He had left the pub at closing time and was walking home alone. As he walked through a children's park he saw something that looked out of place; he could only describe it as a pyramid or a dome-shaped tent or a marquee lit by bright lights. He was struck by the atmosphere of intense quiet around it and he wondered what it was doing there as it looked so odd. Something willed him to go towards it (like a voice inside his head saying the words 'step inside'). He walked into it and it was very bright inside. He then said that it was as if someone had just shredded his memory with scissors. He only remembers waking up the next morning laid on his mother's settee at home wearing his T-shirt, jacket and boots on but with his jeans missing. He said that his jeans were so tight that there was no way that they could be slipped off over his boots. He felt confused and the words 'tent' and 'stepping stones' kept coming into his mind.

Andy was an intelligent, down-to-earth chap and he was a little embarrassed at having to explain such a weird affair. He was worried about what might happen when he was in trance but once he settled into relaxation, I regressed him back to the night in question and he was able to fill in some gaps to his original narrative.

He remembered seeing the marquee with something gaseous ('like dry ice' were his words) around it and a strange colour at the bottom of it. As he was being compelled to walk towards it ('like walking through treacle') he felt the hairs on the back of his neck standing up. As he put his hand on the side of the tent something grabbed hold of him and pulled him onto a stainless-steel-type table. The light was so bright that it hurt his eyes and he tried to fight off whoever or whatever was holding him (he couldn't see them but felt as if there were two of them) as they were tearing at his trousers. He was intensely scared and kicked one of them hard and managed to jump down off the table and run out of the tent, but something even more strange had happened — he was now in a different part of the city. There were lights flashing around the marquee.

As Andy was running, he saw a friend of his coming out of an alleyway and in a shocked voice his friend said 'Christ, where are your strides?' This could only mean that he was already without his jeans ('strides' being a slang word for trousers). His friend backed away and Andy continued running home. Just as an aside, this friend claimed to have been abducted by aliens on that night and later died of a drug overdose having turned to drugs soon after.

He arrived home (having seen a red cloud hovering over a nearby railway bridge) to find the 6 feet high privet hedge outside the house was mysteriously shaking violently. He realised that he didn't have his keys, but as he stood by the back door to the house it opened all by itself and he was lifted up by his elbows by some unseen force and floated through to his sitting room, where he was gently laid down on the settee. He was asking 'who are you?' and 'what do you want?' but all he could remember was hearing a voice in his head saying, 'you're just a boy'. The scissors then came back to cut into his memories and he woke up the next morning when his mum entered the room at 7 a.m. He couldn't remember anything after that and after a while he began to relax and I brought him out of trance.

As you can imagine, Andy was shocked by what he had experienced and relieved that he had at least managed to remember something, especially as it confirmed his feelings that something more had happened that night after he had seen the dome-shaped tent. He contacted me the next day as he was still so surprised at remembering so many strange things; he said when he was in trance the words just came out of his mouth all by themselves and he wanted reassuring that what he'd remembered wasn't simply imagined. Since our session, Andy has occasionally contacted me to tell me that we had opened up 'the door in his mind' behind which the memories were kept and every now and again he receives a bit more information about what happened that night.

On the same night, one of his friends who lived close to another children's park in the city, was awakened in the early hours of the morning by his mother telling him that there was a helicopter flying over the park. He went to look and said that it was not a helicopter but a triangular-shaped space craft with lights around it, which suddenly shot off at high speed and disappeared. His friend said that the weird thing was that as it shot off it made it look as if everything in front of it was moving towards it.

Soon afterwards, Andy noticed that a blood-red mark, like a large pin prick, had appeared on his thigh. He photographed it and blew it up in size to see that it was the shape of a perfect red triangle with perfectly rounded corners. It is still there almost forty years later.

Andy later found out that the date of his experience coincided with the dates of the Rendlesham Forest Incident, which is said to have taken place from 26–28 December 1980. This is a famous series of reported sightings of UFOs in the East of England, close to a US Air Force military base. Over the years he has researched this extensively and is convinced that the beings in his experience are the same ones that were involved at Rendlesham. Although he hasn't been able to recall everything that happened to him that night, he is convinced that he was manipulated by something that was not of this world.

Another strange extraterrestrial regression that I facilitated was with a lady, Kathie, who called me to say that she had been on holiday in a Spanish resort eight or nine years earlier, together with her mother, Edith. Something very strange had happened one night and for the rest of the holiday Edith wouldn't speak to anyone, including Kathie. Soon after they returned home her mother's personality started to change, her mental health declined and since then her mother had never been the same. Kathie was now in her mid-40s and Edith in her early 80s. She explained that since the holiday her formerly perfectly healthy mother had degenerated into a zombie-like state, unable to function and requiring around-the-clock care from family members. Although Kathie had no memory of what had happened, she had a strong sense that it was something to do with aliens. I agreed to regress her back to the night in question to see if we could retrieve any memories.

I should state that when I am doing regression work, I am always cautious not to lead my client or implant anything that could cause me to be accused of leading them in any way. The information should come from the client spontaneously without any suggestions from the therapist. This is especially true of extraterrestrial regressions. I do not agree with the client before or during the regression that what they believe they experienced actually happened. It is possible for a person in trance to make something up and imagine things that are not real, and this is particularly the case if the hypnotist unwittingly (or even knowingly) leads the client or corroborates with them. The therapist should be completely neutral and use what we call 'clean language'. Only after I have observed them in a regression session and heard what they have to say and how they experience it, do I make a judgement as to the veracity of the memories – in other words did they really experience the events from the past or did they just imagine it. There are certain features that I look for during the regressions which indicate to me that it was real or imagined memory.

One common feature of extraterrestrial regressions is that the person who has had the contact with the alien seems to have their conscious memories wiped afterwards, so they are unable to remember anything clearly. However, it appears that they can't wipe the subconscious, which seems to be a deeper store of everything that has ever happened to us; I liken it to a vast computer bank. This means that hypnotic trance is an ideal medium, provided it is done properly and 'cleanly', to unlock or retrieve the consciously forgotten memories.

Kathie turned up at my office pushing Edith in a wheelchair. Kathie had certainly not exaggerated Edith's case as she appeared to be in a total state of dementia, unable to talk or respond to anything we said to her. She sat in her wheelchair with a completely vacant look on her face. Kathie told me in more depth about what had happened to bring her to this appalling state.

They were sharing a room in a hotel complex in a holiday resort. They were enjoying their holiday together and nothing untoward was happening; Edith was happy and relaxed and her normal self. On the night in question, they went to bed in beds that were next to each other, and Kathie fell asleep. At some point during the night, she was awakened by her mother crying out loudly. She saw that the room was full of some type of smoke but there was no smell of burning. Kathie tried to get up out of bed to see if her mother was OK but she said that some force was holding her down and stopping her from getting up. She could hear Edith crying but she couldn't move. She could see two small figures with big heads standing in the room, about a metre and a half tall (four and a half feet) wearing cloaks. After a short time, she blacked out and only woke up the next morning to find Edith asleep in her bed. She had difficulty waking Edith up and when she did, she was confused and couldn't speak coherently. Later that day Edith disappeared for several hours and when she returned, she wouldn't speak. This state of confusion continued for the rest of the holiday and once they arrived back home in the UK she continued to deteriorate mentally into the state that she was now in.

As Kathie shared the story and we talked about it, her mother just sat in her wheelchair saying nothing, occasionally looking around as if trying to understand where she was. Apart from that, even when I tried to talk to her, there was no response to anything we discussed. Obviously, it would be unethical to hypnotise Edith under such circumstances as she was unable to give her consent (and she probably wouldn't have been able to go into hypnosis anyway as she already appeared to be in some form of trance). We had already agreed that it would be best to hypnotise Kathie, to see if she could recall anything other than what she could already consciously remember.

With Edith sitting next to her in the wheelchair, I guided Kathie into hypnosis. Once I'd deepened the trance, I regressed her back to the night in question. After a few minutes, Edith's eyes also closed down and she appeared to go to sleep in her wheelchair. This didn't surprise me as I was talking quietly to her daughter and softly playing gentle relaxation music in the background. Kathie began to talk through her memories of what they did in the hours leading up to the incident. She described their evening meal, getting ready for bed and going to sleep. Just as she was telling me that she was woken up by her mother screaming (and I was hoping that she would be able to recall more details about what had happened), at exactly the same moment as she talked about hearing the screams, suddenly Edith opened her eyes and without warning launched herself upwards and out of her wheelchair. Fortunately, in my sporting years I used to be a goalkeeper, and in a reflex reaction I threw myself forwards too and managed to catch her just before she would have landed face-first on the floor. England football team's goalkeeper would have been proud of the save, although I don't reckon he ever had to throw himself around to catch a little old lady to stop her from being injured. She didn't make a sound as she pushed herself out of the chair.

Picture the scene – Kathie laid in trance in my reclining chair, completely unaware of her mother's escape bid, and me laid half underneath Edith who lay prostrate in my arms on the floor. I was shocked by what had happened, but I managed to lift Edith back into her wheelchair where she promptly fell asleep.

We continued the session as normal, although I kept half an eye on Edith in case she had any more Jack-in-the-box tricks up her sleeve. Unfortunately, Kathie was unable to remember anything else about the incident other than the things she already knew. She was amazed when I told her about her mother jumping out of her wheelchair (she hadn't heard the commotion whilst in trance), and we both agreed that Edith must have been triggered by Kathie talking through the incident and in her own way remembered or relived something that had happened that night. Certainly, it was a most curious action and suggests to me that something very unpleasant took place in that Spanish hotel room that night. Kathie tried to question her but got no response; however she wondered if Edith was perhaps not quite as vegetative as she appeared to be, as she had almost certainly remembered something and had reacted to it in a dramatic and unusual way.

Unfortunately, I was unable to help them further as Kathie had not been able to retrieve any forgotten memories. We were both disappointed but at least Kathie had been given some food for thought. Whatever had happened that night must remain a mystery, but because of Edith's strange and surprising action during the session, I do think that something very significant must have occurred. Whether it was aliens that caused it and subsequently wiped Kathie's memories I cannot say, but I do wonder if Edith experienced something so terrifying that it caused her to lose her mind. Or could it be that the aliens (if it *was* aliens) did something to her mind or her brain that left her without her mental faculties? I asked Kathie to keep in touch with me should her mother start to remember anything or to regain her normal way of life, but I heard nothing.

So, back to my tale, which I mentioned at the start of this chapter, of being featured in the documentary *The Real 4400*. I arrived at a lonely farmhouse in North Yorkshire belonging to Rachel Deveraux and her family. I was not allowed to contact them in advance because the producer of the programme was worried that if I spoke to Rachel beforehand that I might, in some way, implant something into her mind that could contaminate the evidence that might come through during the regression. This was fair enough I thought, as I didn't want to be involved in anything that could spoil the truthfulness of the session. However, I think he was taking it a bit far when as soon as I got out of my car, he started filming me and he didn't let Rachel and I have any time together on our own. Talk about having a suspicious mind!

Rachel was understandably nervous about the whole thing but over a cup of tea in her kitchen (every mouthful dutifully filmed by Mr Suspicious the producer) she told me the family's story.

A few months earlier she, together with her mum and her two sons (aged, I think, around 10 and 11) had been for a meal in a restaurant 20 minutes away from their house. They were driving home after their meal when suddenly they all saw a space craft appear right alongside their car. It was shining bright lights into the car and they all felt an incredible feeling of euphoria. They then remember the spaceship shooting off at high speed and disappearing. They were understandably shocked, but they also felt sad that the UFO had gone. All they could talk about as they drove home was what had happened. As if that wasn't amazing enough, they arrived back at their house to find that the journey which should have taken 20 minutes had taken an hour and 20 minutes. They had lost an hour of their lives and they couldn't account for it. Each of them felt strange and they felt that something else had taken place apart from them just seeing the UFO, but they didn't know what that was. In the weeks after the event, they all became increasingly troubled and upset by not knowing. It was as if they could sense something tangible that was just out of reach of their conscious minds. The boys had started suffering from anxiety attacks and sleep disturbances, including nightmares.

With the TV lights on us and the camera recording the session in her lounge, I took Rachel into trance and regressed her back to the day in question. She firstly talked through leaving the restaurant and getting into the car to drive home, and then she began to remember in more depth the incident:

> *There are bright lights shining all around and into the car and a space ship is alongside us. We're all shocked but I can feel a blissful feeling; I feel euphoric.*

She started to cry but they were tears of happiness. After a few moments she calmed down and continued:

> *They've taken us up in the car to their space craft and we're in a dark room above the earth. I feel happy. There are no walls, just black everywhere; like standing in the middle of space. There's a shield in front with light coming from behind it. I know that there's someone or something on the other side of it, but I can't see what it is. We all stand in a circle facing outwards and holding hands. We're being spoken to telepathically; they're telling me that we are safe and no harm will come to us. There's a big bright light right in front of me, high up. It's watching what the little ones are doing. The small lights are going round and looking at us and talking to each other. There's a big, bright light and smaller lights going around us; floating around us and two smaller lights flying around us, as if they're inspecting us or scanning us. They start with me and the two smaller lights are close to my face and my head; it's as if they're inspecting inside my head. Every time I feel worried the big light comes to my forehead to reassure me telepathically. The two smaller lights are communicating with each other by beams of light; there are no sounds. Now the two lights have moved behind me to inspect the boys. Both of the*

> *boys are laughing, they say it feels like they're being tickled. They think that the boys are funny. The children are laughing, they're really giggling.*

Rachel was smiling and laughing at this point, but then she became anxious as she started to cry.

> *I'm scared for the children but the lights are there and they're telling me that it's fine and they're not going to hurt them; "they're your children". The main light has come back and it's reassuring me.*

Once more she relaxed and let go of the tension. She was silent for a while before she continued:

> *The room is totally dark now but I know that one of the beings is in front of me in the darkness and I'm straining my eyes to see it. It knows that I'm trying to see it. I sense that it's quite small and about two feet in front of me. Now it's totally light again with bright light all around and we're back in the car; we float back down to the ground. The car has also been up in the air, with a road underneath it that doesn't exist. I think we've been about one hundred feet up. Now I'm driving the car with the lights around us and I feel very sad that they have to go. The lights move off very fast and disappear; I feel sad, I didn't want them to go.*

Rachel then talked through some of her conscious memories of driving home with all of them excitedly discussing seeing the lights alongside the car and then shooting off into the distance. She came out of trance both amazed and relieved. She was surprised at the things she had remembered but with a feeling of relief that she now had confirmation that something out of the ordinary had indeed happened on that day; she felt she had some closure on it.

After we finished filming the regression, I was interviewed on camera by the producer who asked me my thoughts about what I had witnessed. I told him that I was 90% convinced that Rachel's memories were true and real. Nowadays, with hindsight, I am 100% convinced. All of the signs I look for in a typical regression session were there, but more than that, I find it very difficult to believe that this 35-year-old woman, her two young sons and her mum were concocting this whole UFO story for some unknown reason. Why would they do that? There were no benefits to going public with the fact they'd had an alien abduction experience. The whole family were emotionally disturbed by not knowing what had happened, and I don't believe that the children (or any of the family) were fabricating things. I believe that they had contact with extraterrestrials that day and would stake my reputation on that being a fact.

My final alien abduction experience in this chapter tells the story of a 15-year-old girl called Ann. She came to me with her mother, Janice, who was very concerned about her daughter's condition. Ann was suffering from anxiety and panic attacks, depression and insomnia. She was so anxious that she was unable to attend school and she also had strange marks on her body. Ann told me that she had vague memories of something happening when she was about 7 years old and since then she had been experiencing psychological problems. She remembered staying at her grandparent's house and waking up one night to see a bright orange glow on the landing outside her room. She got up to have a look and she saw a large orange being with teddy bear-like eyes ('like a hologram' she said). She stood looking at it in awe for a short time before it followed her back into her bedroom. It then jumped, suddenly, and she remembered nothing after that, only waking up in bed screaming hours later. Both Ann and her mum were desperate to find out if anything had happened that night to Ann or was she just imagining things?

I took Ann into hypnosis and once she was deeply in trance I used an age regression technique to guide her back to the night of the alleged incident when she was around 7. Quickly, she began to share with me what she was remembering:

> *I'm playing with my nana and granddad and then nana says it's time for bed. She puts me to bed and turns the light off. Before I fall asleep I look out through the open curtains at the stars and the moon in the sky. Something wakes me up and I see my door is slightly open and there's an orange light shining in from the landing. I get out of bed and open the door and I can see a big light with a man or something in it. It has weird eyes. I'm fascinated; I want to touch it but it won't let me. It comes towards me and I go into my room and close the door and get back into bed. I feel intrigued and a bit scared. It's like a big teddy bear. He walks through the closed door and into my room, then he comes next to me and holds my hand. In my head he's saying that we're going to a happy place, and he holds my hand as I get out of bed and we walk towards the window and the moon and the stars. I see a big red thing in the sky like a ball; it's a weird shape with intricate patterns on it. Why is it there? It doesn't make sense to me. It's like metal but it doesn't look like metal, it's smooth and rounded and it's just floating there. He says that he has to take me and we walk through the wall of the bedroom and we float through the sky into the thing in the sky. We're laughing* (at this point she had a big smile on her face and she was laughing out loud) *and he says that he'll take care of me. I feel confused but happy — I didn't know that we could do this, walk through the air in the sky. We get into the object; he tells me that it's a ship. I can feel that it starts moving.*

Suddenly her face lost its smile and she looked very serious. Her body became tense:

> *He's gone away, he's not there anymore. I feel betrayed; I want him to come back. Now there are three beings coming towards me. They're smaller than him and different; they're the same height as me. They have a different skin colour and their skin is bobbly. They have really interesting, beautiful eyes. They tell me that they're not going to hurt me. They're not talking to me, but sending me thoughts in my head; telling me that I'll be ok. They put me on a big white chair and I can't get out of it. One of them is above me. I feel scared but they're around me telling me that I'll be alright. I'm lying back in the chair (it's like a dentist's chair) and I can see square panels on the ceiling with a mesh on it, though it's all smooth. The floor is blue. I want to go home now; I don't know what is happening. They put a thing like a helmet over my eyes and mouth. I don't like it so I try to take it off but they won't let me. I feel agitated and can see a big, circular light above me and a light like a green laser is going right into my eye. It hurts a lot. I want to get away but I can't move. The laser stops and I can feel them cutting my right hand. It's bleeding but I can't move it. More of them come and they're telling me that I'll be OK but I don't believe them because they're hurting me a lot. They put something gooey in my mouth and I feel funny and happy. I can't stop smiling but I shouldn't be smiling. They put something into my left leg and into my forearm. They look right into my eyes; they're enjoying themselves. I don't want them to leave me but at the same time I want to go home. They're injecting a liquid into my right hand and some of it leaks back out. It hurts but I can't move it. They put a cream or a paste on it and there's no more blood and I can't feel the pain anymore. I ask them why they are doing this and they say it will be better for me — I'll be a new person. They calm me down because I don't like it and*

I feel very vulnerable. The helmet on my head has a disc in it that half covers my eye. They put a big thing from the ceiling into my chest and it sprays stuff into my chest. They're really peaceful and they reassure me that the thing in my hand is a mark so that I'll know. They can't understand why the laser thing in my eye hurts and they take some blood from a vein in my left arm and put something into my head. I get off the chair but I'm very weak so they carry me to another room which is white and silvery with lots of white cushions. They say that it will be time to go back soon but I can rest here for a while. I sleep there but they check up on me every now and again, checking my pulse. When I wake up, I'm back in my bed at my grandparents' house. One of them is sitting on my bed and he reassures me that they'll see me again and everything's fine. Their eyes look weird now and it looks like there's a rip in time and it keeps hitting me in my face. I start screaming and nana comes into my room. I'm dizzy and my head hurts; I feel like I've been somewhere. I don't tell my nana but I can see them behind her walking away, he tells me he's my friend now.

With those words Ann started to stretch and yawn and after a short pause her eyes opened and she came out of trance. It was as if the memories of the incident were over and there was nothing more to remember so her subconscious spontaneously brought her back to full awareness. As you can imagine, both her and her mum were shocked at what had come through in the session, but Ann was also quietly relieved that she now had some reasons as to why she had been so unhappy and stressed for so long. I explained to them that there are many accounts of people who claim to have been taken onto alien space craft and experimented upon, and it appeared that this is what had happened to Ann. I also told them about the idea of implants, which some people believe have been put into them by extraterrestrials. I advised them to do some research and find someone who specialised in removing implants, as it may not have been in Ann's best interests to have them inside her. I'm not sure what happened after this session as neither Ann not Janice kept in touch with me, but at least they had some answers to their questions about Ann's issues. Her experience is certainly unusual and intriguing. It's easy to simply deny that it took place and accuse her of making it all up, but once more (as with Rachel and her family) I question why an intelligent 15-year-old girl would do so. She had nothing to gain by creating such an experience and, for me, all the 'markers' I look for in regression were present, making me feel sure that she wasn't fantasising. I honestly think that she had had an alien abduction experience, and hopefully the regression session helped her to come to terms with it.

Chapter 11

Don't Point That Thing at Me

Christine called me on the phone one day asking for advice. She was a lovely woman, a relatively new Hypnotherapist working in the North of England, and although she hadn't done her initial hypnotherapy training with me, she had attended several of my training courses on specific aspects of therapy. Chris wanted advice about a client whom she had seen a few days earlier.

'He wanted help with his lack of self-confidence', she said. 'I told him when he first contacted me that I could help him with that as hypnotherapy is a very effective way of building confidence. I booked him in for a session and he turned up at my office looking quite shy. He was aged around 40 and once we had talked about his problem I hypnotised him; as he lay in trance I began to use a hypnotic confidence-building suggestion script. All was going well; he lay nicely relaxed, and I was gently feeding his subconscious with the words of the script.

However, after around 15 minutes he slowly began to unzip his flies and he took out his penis and began to masturbate.'

'WHAT?' I shouted, shocked. 'He did WHAT?'

'He took out his dick and started to play with himself.'

There was a pause in the conversation as I tried to take in what she was telling me. I had never heard anything like it before.

'So what happened?'

'Well', she said, 'he just lay there with his eyes closed masturbating.'

'And what did you do?'

'I didn't know what to do, I was just so shocked that I carried on reading my script for another couple of minutes, hoping that he'd put it away.'

'You carried on reading the script, as if nothing was happening?' I asked in amazement.

'Yes, I just didn't know what to do. Nothing like that has ever happened before in a session. After a couple of minutes though, I stopped reading the script and asked him to put his penis away as it wasn't very nice for me.'

'And did he?'

'Yes. He stopped playing with himself and put his dick back in his trousers and zipped himself up and relaxed back into trance again.'

'Right', I said, unsure where all of this was leading. I am used to Hypnotherapists asking me for help, but that is for things like not being sure what to do if the client doesn't go into hypnosis easily, or how to work with a particular issue. But I have never had anyone ask me what to do if they had a sexual pervert in the chair polishing the pickle!

'I continued reading the script and although I was still feeling pretty fazed by things, he seemed to be pretty relaxed, so I kept going. However, after about another ten minutes he did it again.'

'Eh?'

'Yes, he unzipped himself and starting masturbating again. This time he was less quiet about it and as he got more aroused, he started to breathe heavily. I tried to ignore it but...'

'You tried to ignore it?' I said. I was flabbergasted. How on earth could she ignore someone lying in front of her playing with his family jewels?

'So, I stopped reading my script and told him more firmly this time not to do that and to put it away. He stopped and put his dick away, zipped up and relaxed again.'

'What happened then?'

'Nothing else. I finished reading the script and brought him out of trance. I didn't know what to say so I didn't mention it...'

'You didn't mention it?'

'No, I was still shocked and I didn't want to embarrass him. So we finished the session, he paid me, booked another session next week and left.'

'He booked another session?' I was incredulous.

'Yes', she said sheepishly. 'He said he wanted to see me again.'

I was silent again for a while, still staggered by what she had told me.

'What should I have done?' she asked.

'What you should have done', I replied forcefully, 'as soon as he took his penis out was to stop reading, tell him to put it away and open his eyes. You should have picked up the phone and told him that if he didn't leave you immediately that you would call the police. You should have started to dial 999 and told him to go out of your door as fast as his three legs could carry him. Didn't you think about the danger that you could have been in?'

'I did afterwards, when I'd had chance to think about it', she said. 'But at the time I was still astonished at what was happening; it was so outrageous that I didn't know how to handle it.'

I went on: 'And if he had tried to tell you that he didn't know what he was doing because he was in trance, you just tell him that's bullshit, and he was just getting off on one. Nobody does anything like that in hypnosis without knowing exactly what they are doing.'

'Yes, I know', she said quietly.

I was trying not to tell her off, but she had completely mishandled the situation and as a woman working on her own in her office she could have been in a very dangerous position. She had to realise the gravity of the situation.

'So, what you need to do now is to call him and cancel the appointment, tell him that what he did was completely disgusting and that if he contacts you again you'll go to the police and report him.'

'I've already done that Steve; I called him earlier and told him that I was not prepared to see him again.'

'And what did he say', I asked.

'He said that he was disappointed as he'd enjoyed the session' (I'm sure he did, I thought to myself) 'but he wanted me to reconsider as he felt that he still needed help with his lack of confidence.'

'And what did you do, Chris?'

'I told him "no" but I gave him your number and recommended that he comes to see you.'

Long Pause ... 'er, thanks Chris'.

Chapter 12

Three, Two, One, You're Back in the Room (or, Maybe Not)

Sam was a fellow Hypnotherapist who was coming to me for therapy. I see a lot of therapists who come to work on their own issues, and I am a total advocate for all therapists having therapy. Unfortunately, this doesn't happen as often as I think it should, as many therapists have the attitude that their clients may need therapy, but they themselves don't. What this means is that they are not as balanced emotionally or psychologically as they would like to have you believe. It's said that only 4% of people are truly balanced and functional, and therapists are no different from everyone else in this regard. Although we all carry emotional pain within us, if that emotional pain is severe your therapist will not be as functional or grounded as you would like. Many therapists are carrying a lot of emotional baggage and although these 'Wounded Healers' may have a lot of compassion for their fellow man as a result of their own suffering, they may not be able to offer the client a truly open and impartial space in which to work. They may sometimes get triggered when a client is sharing their feelings, and they may give advice (which therapists should never do, by the way. My mentor, Wilf Proudfoot, used to say 'NEVER give advice') which is misleading and biased, coming from their reactiveness to a client's pain. I read of a psychotherapist in the United States years ago who would get her clients to leave home and move in with her if they were having a bad time. Talk about *severely* misplaced boundaries!

Anyway, back to Sam, who wanted to heal his emotional 'stuff' so that he would be a better role model for his clients. He turned up one morning for his session and started to tell me about what had happened at a therapists' peer supervision meeting he had attended the night before. This was a meeting of local Hypnotherapists in his area who got together once a month to discuss therapy topics, share ideas and therapy techniques etc. He said that there were about 12 therapists there who usually attended, and also a new therapist whom nobody had seen before. Sam said that the new man was very quiet and didn't join in with any of the conversations. He just sat in the corner looking troubled. After a while, the host of the meeting apologised to the man for not asking him to introduce himself at the start of the meeting. However, would he like to say a few words to the group about himself, his training and his therapy practice? The man shuffled in his chair for a few moments and slowly started to talk. His voice was monotone and he appeared to be very unhappy. He told the group that he had only recently completed his hypnotherapy training and only seen one client. The reason he had come to this meeting was because of what had happened in that first client session. He was seriously considering giving up being a therapist because of it.

He was quiet for a few moments and the host told him that one of the things that was often discussed at these meeting were problems with clients as some of the more experienced therapists could give advice. The man began to tell his story.

His first client was an 80-year-old man who was feeling anxious and having panic attacks. He said that he listened to the client give information about himself and his anxieties before he told him a little about hypnosis and how it could help. When this was done, he took him into hypnosis and began to deepen the trance. As this was his very first client session, he was nervous but felt that he had managed to hide his nerves and he was relieved when the client had closed his eyes and began to relax. He said that the man had gone into trance easily and so he then started to read a script to the client which was all about letting go of anxiety. The aim was to implant suggestions into his client's subconscious to help him to feel calmer. All was going well, the client was deeply relaxed and very still (usually a sign of deep trance), he was starting to feel more confident as he read through the script, and he hoped that his words would have a positive effect on the old man in the coming days. After about 40 minutes he had finished reading his suggestions and he started to count the client out of trance. This is a usual process for many hypnosis sessions; when we are ready to bring the client back to conscious awareness, we count up from one to ten, asking them to open their eyes on the number ten. However, the old man was obviously very deep as he didn't come back. Sometimes this happens, and also some clients are enjoying the relaxation so much that they don't want to come back. He said that when he did his training, he was taught that if the client doesn't come back out of trance when they are counted out, to do the count out again but this time in a louder voice and with more energy. This he did, speaking much louder (also he wondered if the man was a little hard of hearing because of his age or if he had even fallen asleep) but once more, on the number ten and being given the instruction to open his eyes the man carried on relaxing. Maybe he was asleep he thought, so this time as he counted to ten in an even louder voice, he tapped the sides of the chair to gently wake him up. It was at this point that he realised that the old man was not moving and was, in fact, dead.

You can imagine the shock of the therapists in the room as they heard this. His very first client! No wonder he was wondering whether to carry on in his new career. He found out afterwards that the old man had heart problems and had just simply passed away in the chair; it was nothing that he had done that had caused this but as you can imagine he still felt terrible. The therapists did their best to reassure him that this sort of thing never happens and that he was just incredibly unlucky, but Sam didn't know whether their words were enough to convince him. All you can say, I suppose, is that at least the old man had a quiet and beautiful passing. I can think of worse ways to die.

Chapter 13
The Power of Tapping

I walked into my office one morning and listened to a gloriously vague and exciting message on my answerphone that had been left the night before:

'Hi Steve, it's Doreen here. You don't have to call me back, but you might like to know that the tapping you did on me last year has saved my life and the lives of five children. Bye.'

Don't have to call me back! Who did she think I was?

Doreen had come to me a year earlier, suffering from a severe phobia of the sea. She was about to go on holiday abroad and she wanted to join her husband when he went into the sea and take part in normal beach activities. Whenever she was on a beach she could stand at the edge of the water, but as soon as the sea covered her feet she would start panicking and run out of the water. In our session we had spent an hour doing EFT (Emotional Freedom Technique) or 'tapping' as it is more colloquially known and at the end of the session she didn't feel frightened when she thought of being in the water on her forthcoming holiday. I assumed her phobia had been fixed but didn't hear anything else from her, until the answerphone message on this morning.

When I rang her back, she told me that the work we had done had indeed shifted the phobia. On holiday she had not just been paddling in the sea but after a couple of days she was able to swim on her back! Then, she began to tell me how EFT had actually saved lives.

A few weeks earlier she was walking along Cleethorpes beach in the UK with her grandchildren and their friends (ranging in age from 4 to 11) when they became cut off from the main beach as the tide came in behind them at speed in a pincer movement. Realising that they were caught, they could only watch in growing trepidation as the water rose higher and higher around them and the area of sand they were standing on became smaller and smaller. Unbeknown to them, this area is a known danger spot and the coastguards are always monitoring it in case people get trapped in this way. The coastguards had sent out a rescue boat to try to save them, but Doreen and the children were unaware of this. All they could see was the seawater closing in on them (Doreen found out afterwards that because of the speed of the incoming tide on that day the rescue launch would not have got to them in time).

As the children became increasingly frightened, Doreen decided that they had to try to escape. Telling them not to panic, she picked up the youngest child in her arms and together they all began moving through the water. They had difficulty walking as they were wading through thick, muddy sand which kept sucking their feet down, but they kept pushing on as the water got higher around them. Doreen wondered, as the water came over her waist to her chest, if they were going to make it, but eventually they reached dry land and safety.

'I know for a fact', she told me, 'that if we hadn't have done the tapping session last year that we would all be dead now. There is absolutely no way that I would have dared to go into such deep water. I used to be so terrified of sea water and I know we would have just stood on that sand bank, panicking as we watched the water getting closer to us, before we were swept out to sea. The tapping session you did with me saved our lives.'

It was an amazing story, but is only one of many thousands from people around the world whose lives have been transformed by using this simple technique (check out the EFT Introductory Video on YouTube if you want to be convinced). So, what is EFT, I hear you ask?

Emotional Freedom Technique is a process that involves tapping with the fingertips on various points on the body whilst the client tunes into their problem. They repeat various phrases to help them stay focussed on the issue (and the emotional and physical feelings which it engenders) and the aim is to neutralise or soften the negative feelings or thoughts which the presenting problem has been causing. Often this happens in a single session.

It can work on a wide range of issues, including phobias, anxieties and panic attacks; addictive cravings (food, cigarettes, alcohol, chocolate, drugs); physical issues and pain; PTSD; and Irritable Bowel Syndrome to name just a few. Therapists who learn EFT usually use it on anything and everything.

It is often referred to as 'psychological acupuncture' (except that it doesn't use needles) and is one of a group of therapies known as Energy Therapies as they work on the sub-molecular energy pathways (known as meridians) throughout the body. Whereas acupuncture uses these same meridians but has limited success with problems of a psychological nature, EFT works highly effectively on such issues. It appears that tapping on the various points around the body (the head, face, chest, under arm and fingers) realigns the subtle energies and allows them to flow freely, thus releasing the blocked or locked-in feelings which have been causing the problem. EFT has an extremely high rate of success (usually 50 – 80%) and it also empowers the client as many EFT practitioners teach their clients the tapping system so that they can use it whenever the need arises.

One of my clients was cured in minutes of her cravings for alcohol (so much so that the thought of a glass of wine disgusted her) and another lost her chocolate addiction so completely that she didn't have a desire for chocolate for eighteen months after a ten-minute tapping session. On an EFT training course that I ran in the UK some years ago, one of the therapists on the course, a 30-something year old woman, sat in obvious pain listening to my explanation of the tapping system. I had noticed her at the start of the course as she held her body very stiffly. If she wanted to look to the side she turned her whole body and not just her neck, and at one point she dropped her pen on the floor and instead of bending down to pick it up she had to go down onto her knees with her back straight and pick it up from the side with one of her hands. I asked for someone with pain to volunteer themselves so I could demonstrate the technique on them, and she offered herself straight away.

In front of the group she explained her problem. Five years earlier she had contracted a mystery virus which had hospitalised her for months and nearly killed her. Since then she had been unable to move or bend her upper body or turn her neck. The whole upper part of her body was rigidly locked tight and she was in constant pain. Even trying to bend over or turn her neck produced excruciating pain. We began doing some general (called 'global') tapping on the pain and after a few minutes the pain level had dropped substantially, from nine out of ten to four out of ten. However, her body was still rigidly stuck and her neck would not move so I began tapping and asking her to focus on the emotions that her body was holding onto from the time she had spent in hospital. These included the trauma of nearly dying, of worrying about her children and how they would cope without her, as well as being helpless whilst she lay in a hospital bed. After a few rounds of tapping whilst she tuned into the deeper elements of her illness, she was able to start turning her neck and to bend over a little. She was not cured, but her body was starting to let go of the locked-in traumas which it had been holding onto. I sensed that there was some anger somewhere in her that she was not letting go of, and it was when I asked her to think about this that she talked about the worst part of her experience. At the time of her illness she ran her own successful hairdressing salon, and whilst she was in hospital two of the stylists who worked for her offered to run the business for her and keep it going until she was well enough to return to work. She trusted them as friends but during the months she was in hospital they ran the business dry, stealing money and equipment from her so that eventually there was no business left and she went bankrupt. The betrayal of this was the core of the problem and as we tapped on her anger she became, in turn, furious, then emotional, then finally calm. We had spent only around ten minutes tapping but she slowly started to turn her neck and bend her back. The pain had completely gone and so had the physical stiffness and rigidity. She could turn her neck easily and freely and even bend over and touch her toes. It was as though she had never had a problem in the first place. She was so amazed that her physical problems were healed that she began dancing around the room, bending over and turning her neck and crying with delight. The other group members who had seen her living a half-life during the previous months, hardly able to move and in constant pain just sat applauding and crying. Talk about a miracle cure — I felt like Jesus!

I remember another training course in which I was demonstrating the EFT technique on a lady who had a phobia of driving. She was able to drive her car but she felt scared whenever she was driving (when I asked her to score them she said that the feelings of fear could get as high as nine out of ten when she was on the road). I asked her to tune into the fear by imagining that she was sitting in her car driving at that moment, and after only 30 seconds of tapping the fear had completely evaporated. It was as fast as that. She just knew that she wasn't frightened anymore after only 30 seconds of tapping. It seemed too good to be true so to test if the phobia had truly been eradicated, I asked her to take me for a drive in her car in the lunch break. I sat in her passenger seat as she drove around town without a care in the world; the phobia was indeed no more. Unfortunately, what I hadn't anticipated was that she was the world's worst driver. I sat in the passenger seat terrified as she drove so badly that I thought I was going to be killed. We got back to the course venue and I was shaking – I had to do some tapping to de-traumatise myself before I could continue teaching!

On yet another EFT training course, this time one which I was running in Stavanger, Norway, one of the members of the course, a Hypnotherapist called Helen, 'phoned me on the first day of the course to say that she was too ill to attend. She had been in hospital for several days suffering from kidney stones. In hospital a CT scan showed that she had a lot of them and she was in excruciating pain. Painkillers were not helping and she had had very little sleep for a week or so. She was now at home waiting for the next stage in her treatment from the hospital. She was disappointed that she was unable to attend the training course as she was looking forward to learning EFT so she could use it with her clients. I called her the next day to see how she was feeling and she told me that there had been no change in her condition, so I asked her if she wanted to come to the course that day so I could demonstrate EFT on her in front of the rest of the students. I said that I was hopeful that EFT could help to reduce the pain she was in. As she was desperate for anything that could help, Helen agreed to take part in the demonstration.

When she arrived she looked dreadful; she was walking with an effort and she looked exhausted and drained. She told me that the pain level at that time had a score of eight out of ten; a few days earlier it had been ten out of ten but the painkillers were just taking the edge off it. I started tapping on her, asking her to repeat my words as I tapped on the EFT points around her body. Initially I just did 'global tapping' on the pain but it had no effect, so I then began to tap on the emotional causes of the kidney stones. Helen told me a little about her dysfunctional childhood with difficult parents, and so as I tapped on the points, she verbalised her feelings about her childhood. Her Inner Child felt so very angry. In my experience kidney stones are like chunks of unreleased anger and so we tapped extensively on this anger. The pain level started to drop, to four out of ten, to two out of ten, and after an hour of tapping on many aspects of her childhood it was down to one out of ten. She looked amazed (so did most of the group who were watching the demo) and incredibly relieved. I taught her the basic tapping system and asked her to continue the tapping in the coming days at home. She left looking like a new woman, looking forward to catching up on her lost sleep.

On its own, that would be a tremendous success, but what happened next was nothing short of miraculous. Helen called me a couple of days later to say that the pain had almost gone. However, she had spent most of the night after our session (which had taken place on the Saturday) sitting on the toilet with blood pouring out of her. She had experienced no pain and she had not panicked, as she knew that her body was releasing something as a result of the EFT session. Today (Monday) she had gone to the hospital for her appointment with the specialist to discuss surgery, but her new scan showed that there was not a single stone left in her body! Her consultant was shocked and couldn't believe how such a thing could have happened. In less than a week since he had first seen her, she was completely free of kidney stones. Helen tried to explain to him about the EFT session but he just fobbed it off as nonsense (the standard medical line when a doctor is presented with something that doesn't fit with his or her rigid mind set is that there has been a 'spontaneous remission' so they don't have to look more carefully at the possible causes that would question their inflexible view of the world). She knew, though, that EFT had cured her body of its illness. I have seen Helen several times over the years since our session, and not only have the kidney stones never returned but also she feels much better about her childhood.

EFT grew out of an earlier energy therapy linked to kinesiology, namely TFT (Thought Field Therapy), an extremely effective, if slightly cumbersome, range of tapping procedures developed in the USA by Dr Roger Callahan. An early TFT practitioner was an American engineer called Gary Craig who felt that TFT was too complicated. Using his engineering background he took TFT apart and re-assembled it in the much simpler form of EFT.

Gary has continued to devote his life to the development of EFT and has refined the technique over the years. In 2003 I was honoured to be a member of a group of 15 therapists from around the world invited to his home in the States to help him develop a new way of working with EFT. At one stage, Gary worked with me on a disturbing memory from my childhood (which I had not realised held such a deep emotional charge) and blew away its effects completely. Words cannot describe the feeling of freedom that I felt. All the locked-in feelings from the memory poured out to be replaced by a free flow of positivity and joy.

What I'm leading up to here, in writing about EFT, is one of the biggest and most satisfying therapy successes in my career.

Sally called me to ask if I could help her daughter, who was experiencing what she called 'night terrors'. She had a strange tale to tell. Every evening for the past six or seven months she had put her 2[1]/2-year-old daughter Poppy to bed at 6 p.m. Poppy was laid in her cot and Sally or her husband would talk or sing her to sleep. Every night though, at around 6.40 p.m., they would hear Poppy screaming in terror. They would rush upstairs and it would take about 40 minutes to calm her down. They didn't know why she was doing this but they were obviously worried about her and stressed because they didn't know what to do to help her.

I explained to Sally that Poppy was too young for me to use hypnosis on her (usually children from about 7 years' old and upwards are suitable for hypnotherapy) but that I would use EFT, an unusual tapping process to see if it would help. Sally sounded sceptical but as she was desperate, she agreed to bring Poppy to see me.

They arrived for the session; Poppy was a cute little girl who wouldn't leave mummy's arms because she didn't understand where she was or what was happening. She looked at me shyly through her beautiful big eyes, and quickly hid her face whenever she caught me looking or smiling at her. Sally told me in more depth about the weird nightly routine that was spoiling their lives.

She said that each night when Poppy woke up screaming, they would find her standing up in her cot, her body rigid and her arms outstretched as she stared at a particular spot high up on the wall. She was fixated on this one spot and couldn't seem to tear her eyes away from it. She would be so distressed that it would take them around 40 minutes to pull her attention away from the wall, and to calm her down enough so that she would eventually go back to sleep. Why it happened at almost exactly 6.40 each evening Sally did not know. They had checked for any sounds or noises inside or outside the house but there was nothing. They had never allowed her to watch any scary TV or read any scary stories to her. They were very focussed on making sure that in the hours leading up to bedtime Poppy was cared for and in a calm environment.

What made it even more odd is that several nights each week, at around 12.40 a.m., Poppy would awaken screaming again; her body rigid with fear, her arms outstretched and stiff and her eyes fixated on the same place on the wall. Each time this happened it would take about 20 minutes to calm her down and get her off to sleep. Sally said that she and her husband were quite exhausted by the whole situation and unable to live a normal home life because of it.

I asked a few questions about Poppy's life experiences, but there were no traumas that Sally could report. Her relationship with her husband was settled and very loving with no arguments or shouting around the house between the two of them. Poppy's birth had been a little bit stressful but whilst Sally had been carrying her there had been no traumas in Sally's life that could have affected Poppy whilst in the womb. I explained to Sally about the tapping procedure, and she was intrigued to know how tapping on points on the body could possibly help Poppy to let go of her night terrors. She was even more intrigued when I told her that I wasn't going to tap on Poppy, but on her.

I used a technique known as 'surrogate tapping', in which as Sally held Poppy in her arms, I tapped on Sally whilst she said various words and phrases as if she was Poppy. The concept behind this is that if two people are touching each other, they form one energy field. So by doing EFT on Sally it was actually affecting Poppy. I 'fluffed' (my therapist's word for 'improvised') a lot of phrases that just came into my head as I tapped around the points on Sally's head, face, chest and hands, asking her to say the words as if she was her daughter. Poppy watched all of this through eyes of wonder, not saying anything but listening to everything we said as I tapped. Occasionally I tapped a couple of times gently on Poppy and then went back to tapping on her mum. I cannot remember what I said as I tapped as most of it just came into my head like a stream of free association, but I do remember talking about birth trauma as I tapped around. At one point Sally became quite emotional (which was surprising as all of the statements I was making were about Poppy) but apart from that nothing dramatic happened. I spent maybe 20 to 30 minutes tapping and felt that we had done enough for that session. I asked to see them again in a few weeks' time, as by that time Sally would know if the work we had done had had any positive effect. Obviously, we couldn't tell if I'd been successful as Poppy was unable to tell us how she felt; she just gazed at me in silence and then waved goodbye as she went out of the door.

Sally came back with Poppy three weeks later, and as she arrived she couldn't wait to tell me how things had been since I'd seen them. 'It's been like a miracle!' she said excitedly. 'We haven't had one single episode since we've seen you. Every night Poppy has gone to bed at her usual time and has slept through till the next morning. Only on one night did she wake up at 12.40, but she was only crying a little and we soon got her back to sleep. We can't believe the difference; it's just incredible.'

I was so pleased to hear this, but before I could say anything Sally carried on: 'But more than that, Poppy has changed dramatically too. The staff working at her nursery have been asking us what we've done to her as she's changed so much. She now has so much more confidence than before; she used to spend a lot of time on her own but now she's playing all day long with the other children. She's interacting with everyone. They say that it's like having a different child there. And even more than that, her hair is now growing properly. Ever since she was born her hair wasn't growing much, but now it's growing normally. It's been like a miracle!'

As you can imagine I was so pleased that we'd such a wonderful result. This little girl could now live a normal life without all the fears she had inside her. I still don't know what caused her night terrors, but something we tapped on had been released and she was now free of them. Little Poppy again didn't say anything but she did nod or shake her head this time when I spoke to her, and she was a lot brighter than the first time I'd seen her. Apparently, a few hours before they came to this second appointment Poppy had asked Sally 'are we going to see my friend Steven tonight?'

We did a little bit more tapping just to make sure that I'd covered all of the possible aspects of the problem and after a big hug from Sally and a little hug from Poppy they said goodbye with Poppy waving and smiling at me as they left my office.

Several months later I walked into my office in the morning to find Sally had left an answerphone message the night before:

'Hi Steve, it's Sally here; you may remember you treated Poppy a few months ago. Poppy has been completely fine since we saw you. I'm just calling to tell you that it's seven o'clock in the evening and my husband and I are sitting down to enjoy a nice relaxing meal with a glass of wine. We couldn't have done this before we saw you. I just wanted to say thank you so much for what you've done.'

With a smile on my face, a tear in my eye and a lump in my throat, and the vision of a lovely little girl waving at me as she left my office smiling, I sat down at my desk and readied myself for my first client of the new day.

Chapter 14

Be Afraid. Be Very Afraid.

I guess that seeing that you've got this far into the book it hopefully means that you're enjoying the read (and that you're not just flicking through the pages in a book shop wondering whether to buy it), in which case if you continue reading the rest of this chapter you may end up not sleeping well tonight and keeping the lights on at home all night.

This is because I'm going to share with you an aspect of therapy that doesn't happen very often, but having said that it happens more often than you would expect — namely spirit attachments. I realise that probably sounds scary, and in Erica's case it certainly was. She was a 13-year-old girl whose mum, Diane, called me sounding very concerned about her daughter:

'It's as though sometimes she's just not there', she said, 'she just goes "distant" and we can't get her back for a while. She's also very forgetful, and it's as if her brain doesn't work all of the time. She's even had a brain scan. Apparently, there's nothing wrong with her brain but her brainwaves are not quite normal.'

Although I wasn't sure if I could help her, as the problem seemed an odd one, I told Diane that I'd see Erica as I know from experience that once we start working in hypnosis the subconscious is able to work on issues in its own way and can often create a resolution to even the most indissoluble of problems. And as the process is usually fast, we would know very quickly whether I could help or not.

They arrived at my office one evening and Erica seemed a typical teenager, although she sounded quite 'down' in herself when she explained her symptoms. She had been feeling odd for over a year, sometimes feeling dizzy and quite often disassociating from the world around her. Once when she was at a children's playground she felt that she didn't know who she was or where she was. She also felt anxious a lot of the time and she had started to bite her nails, and she didn't like being on her own — if she were alone in a room she would feel scared.

I was beginning to wonder if Erica's problem was an anxiety state that was manifesting these symptoms, but it was what she said next that made me wonder if something more sinister was going on. She said that she often felt that something or somebody was inside her, and that this something or somebody would talk to her and tell her things. Sometimes if she looked at herself in a mirror, she thought she could see someone half inside and half outside her. I didn't tell either Erica or her mum my suspicions as I didn't want to scare them or be accused of leading Erica in some way, but my immediate thought when she said this was that Erica could have a spirit or spirits attached to her.

Let me explain this in more depth. It appears that when someone dies their soul or spirit leaves the physical body and travels upwards to the spirit realms, where it meets with other souls who have been around it for many incarnations (its 'Soul Group'). It also goes through a process of learning and healing and renewal, ready for its next life. The concept of reincarnation is an ancient one and is the basis for Past Life Therapy. For more information on this subject I recommend Michael Newton's brilliant book *Journey of Souls*. Newton does all of his regression sessions in the time in between lives, and his subjects come up with fascinating and similar stories of what happens in the afterlife.

However, sometimes upon the death of the physical body the spirit doesn't go on this journey and stays around on earth. The reasons for this can be many and varied — sometimes they are lost or confused, especially if they have had a sudden, unexpected death and don't know where to go; sometimes they are scared, especially if they have a lot of guilt in them from things that they have done in their lives and they fear they will be judged or they will go to Hell (which as a result of the thousands of regression sessions that I've facilitated I believe doesn't exist by the way); sometimes they want to stay around loved ones on earth; sometimes they are angry and want to stay around people who have harmed them whilst they were alive and try to cause them problems. What the spirit of the dead person often does is attach itself to someone close by in order to feel safe. It usually connects with someone's energy field, although sometimes it connects with their body and can cause physical problems. The person who is carrying the spirit then picks up on its energies and becomes influenced by the negative feelings of the spirit. If the spirit is unhappy or sad the person may feel depressed; if the spirit is angry or scared the person will feel these feelings.

When I first heard of the concept of spirit attachment at the start of my career, I thought it was a load of baloney, and that any client who thought they had a spirit attached to them was making something up to give them an excuse as to why they had emotional or psychological issues. Once I spoke to more experienced colleagues though, I began to change my attitude to a more open one. These colleagues (who were quite rational and down-to-earth people) had experienced spirit attachments with their clients and they told me stories that began to convince me as to the possible reality of it. To give the subject a gloss of respectability, I came upon the book *The Unquiet Dead* by Dr Edith Fiore. She was an American psychologist who, after some years working in traditional ways using traditional psychology procedures, was opened up to the possibility that some of her clients had attachments. She then worked regularly with spirit release, in which as a result of a particular protocol she helped her clients to release the spirits and to send them 'home', to where they should have gone when they died. The clients subsequently became cured of the issues for which they had sought her help.

As a result of Dr Fiore's book and discussions with experienced colleagues, I would occasionally, when my client was in trance, ask their subconscious if they had any spirit attachments. I would do this by using the Ideo-Motor Response (you may remember this is the 'yes/no' finger signal that I set up with my client's subconscious) and ask the subconscious if they had any spirits attached to their body or their aura. I would only usually do this if, when I was asking the subconscious to indicate the cause of their problem, it responded that there were no emotional traumas causing the problem. Obviously, the client's problem had to come from somewhere as we don't catch a phobia or a depression or an anxiety state by sitting on the bus next to someone who passes it on to us like flu. If there were no emotional causes from the past in this present life, from previous lifetimes or that we have inherited from our ancestors, I would then ask the subconscious if there were any spirits attached to my client which were causing the phobia or depression etc. If the finger responded with a 'yes' I would go through my spirit release process and in most cases the spirit would leave within a few minutes. As a result my client's problems would usually cease or be radically reduced.

Curiously enough, you would expect that if my client was a believer in the afterlife and spirits and the like, that their finger would rise to say 'yes', but that wasn't always the case. I have regularly had 'left-brain' people who have no such beliefs who found they had spirit attachments. I remember one highly successful businessman, a director of several companies, lying in my chair in trance in his expensive suit, buttoned up shirt and tie, releasing a spirit that had caused him to be depressed for many years. It appears he had picked it up in hospital, when he had been very worried about undergoing a major operation (apparently hospitals are good places to pick up spirits as hospitals have many dead people in them!).

One of the most convincing stories I heard about spirit attachments came from my friend Ray, who was a very level-headed chap who had an interest in spiritual matters and the paranormal. He told me that when he was in his 20s he had a girlfriend, Anne, who was practising hands-on healing and who was also a trance medium. This meant that she would go into trance when in a circle of spiritual people and allow dead people to speak through her to their loved ones. Ray wasn't totally sure about the reality of these things but was very open-minded and so he went along with Anne to her healing group in a church hall in the Midlands every week. The healers there invited him to practise his own healing abilities (apparently we all have such abilities) and helped him to develop them. After a while he was an accepted part of the team of healers, and each week would work with different people who had physical problems. He then told me about his experience which proved to him that spirit attachment is a reality.

He said that he was with Anne at their healing group and that during the evening he spotted a young man in his early 20s who slipped into the hall and sat at the back of the room observing proceedings. The man looked very nervous and was constantly twitching and jerking and rubbing his hands around his face and head. However, he didn't come up for healing but just sat at the back of the room. The healers were at the front of the hall working in pairs on people who were sitting in chairs with their eyes closed. At the end of the evening, Ray went over to him and asked him if he'd like to receive some healing. As he got closer to him, Ray could see that he was trembling and was obviously very anxious. The man declined but asked Ray if he could ask him a few questions because he felt really bad. By this stage Ray had been joined by his girlfriend, Anne, and they listened to the man's story. He said that his name was Pete and that until recently he had been a soldier in the British army stationed in Afghanistan. He had been involved in several hostile incidents in which he been under fire and had seen some of his comrades injured or killed. Since the worst incident, in which his best pal was shot and killed right next to him, he had been suffering from severe anxiety. He was shaking all the time and felt scared and panicky for no reason.

Just as he was reaching this point in his story, my friend Ray was startled when a man's voice suddenly came out of Anne's mouth and loudly shouted 'Pete'. Ray turned in shock and saw that Anne's eyes had closed down and her head slumped forwards on her chest. She was standing in trance! Ray looked back at the soldier who was standing looking at Anne with a look of shock on his face. Again the man's voice came out of Anne's mouth: 'Pete. Pete. It's me, Terry.'

'Terry?' said the soldier, 'Is that you?'

'Yes', said Anne, or whoever it was that was speaking through her. 'It's me, Terry. What's happened? Where am I? What's going on?'

Ray stood in amazement and watched and listened to a three-way conversation that was going on, with only two people involved.

'Terry', said Pete, the soldier, 'you can't be here, you're dead. You died. You died in the ambush.'

'I don't know where I am. Pete, I'm scared, what's happening?'

By this stage some of the other healers had joined the scene and one of them had previous experience with this sort of bizarre event. He gently asked Pete who Terry was and what had happened to him. Pete said that Terry was his best mate in the battalion. During a vicious incident in Afghanistan in which they were together under heavy enemy fire, Terry had been killed instantly by a bullet as he stood next to Pete. Pete had been devastated by the loss of his best pal and ever since then had suffered from what he thought was severe PTSD. However, as the healer now explained, what had happened was that Terry had died so quickly that he was confused and afraid as he left his body. He had immediately hooked into Pete because he was familiar with Pete's energy; the trouble is Pete was then able to feel Terry's fear and bad feelings and these were manifesting themselves in the form of Pete's anxiety state.

The healer then spoke to Terry, through Anne, telling him that he was now dead and that he had connected to Pete because they were friends. However, Terry had to move on now and leave Pete and go to the place where we all go when we die, a place of love and healing. As the healer continued to talk to the spirit of Terry and give it instructions of how to go, Anne started to jerk as though something was leaving her body. Once this was done Anne slowly came out of trance and opened her eyes. Pete, although totally shocked, was much calmer and the bad feelings that he had turned up with were no longer there. Terry's spirit had been sent 'home' and Pete was freed of the anxieties which had been causing him so much trouble. Not surprisingly, my friend Ray had also become an instant convert to the concept of spirit attachments!

As you can imagine, hearing such a story from a reliable first-hand source persuaded me to become more open-minded towards the concept of spirit attachments.

So, when I took Erica into trance (Diane stayed in the room to watch the session as Erica was nervous about it) and her subconscious took control of a finger on her left hand, I asked if there were any emotional traumas in the past that were causing the strange feelings that she had been experiencing. The finger rose to say 'yes'. Although there were no traumas in this present life, there were some in her past lives and in her ancestor's lives. I then asked if she had any spirit attachments and the finger shot up in the air to say 'yes'. It next said that there were several spirits. I looked at Diane, who looked back at me and nodded. I then began going through my spirit release procedure, and after a few minutes Erica's subconscious indicated that most, but not all, of the spirits had gone. It appeared that there were two spirits left that were stubbornly refusing to go. Throughout most of this Erica was just allowing things to happen, but then as she lay with her eyes closed, she told me that she could 'see' a little boy next to her and that his name was Edward. It's unusual for my clients to see a spirit as most of them just feel something or some energy leaving them, but in this case Erica was visualising the spirit of a child that had become connected to her. With this information I was able to send Edward onwards, but Erica's IMR finger indicated that there was still one more spirit that hadn't gone. She screwed up her face and slowly pointed towards the bookshelves in my office. 'I can see a man, dressed all in black, standing over there by the bookshelves', she said quietly. She started to shake a little and she said that her face was tingling. I felt the room go cold. A shiver ran up my spine. 'He's got black hair and he's wearing a long black coat and he's running his fingers over the books.'

I then continued to go through my spirit release instructions but the man in black wouldn't go. He just stayed standing by my bookshelves, and the room continued to feel very cold. After a few minutes Erica told me that he had walked out of the door, but I wasn't sure if he had gone 'home' or not. We had come to the end of the session so I brought Erica out of trance. She was perplexed at what had happened but she felt a lot calmer in herself and lighter inside. Diane told me that she was not surprised at all; in fact (and she hadn't said this to Erica) she had heard of such things before and she had wondered if Erica had some spirit attachments. This was a relief to me as I had half expected her to demand what the hell had been going on. They made another appointment for a couple of weeks later and left my office, Erica with a smile on her face.

I started to tidy up the room and was analysing the session in my mind when I noticed that the room was still cold. I checked to see if the central heating was on — it was. I started to sense that something in the office was not right. It always had a gentle and light energy of calmness; now it actually felt heavy, dull and threatening. I always pride myself on being a level-headed chap and not prone to giving in to weird imaginings, but I could have sworn that someone else was in the room with me. It felt as though I was being watched. I'm not a psychic so I didn't know if it was my imagination or if there really was a spirit in the office with me. Maybe one of Erica's spirit attachments hadn't gone properly into the light? Or could it be the man in black was still there?

I told myself not to be silly and carried on tidying up and left the room. In those days I was living and working in a private house in the Yorkshire town of Beverley, and as we had finished the session quite late it was around 10 o'clock when I went up to my bedroom. I did a bit of reading before I went to bed but I couldn't shake off the feeling that someone was watching me. I was doing my best not to feel spooked but struggled to feel at ease. I went to bed and had a restless night. The feeling of being watched and the room being cold continued all of the next day, so I phoned Alan, a friend who classed himself as an 'ex-white witch' and who was very experienced with ghostly matters (he was often called upon to clear haunted houses of their ghosts). He tuned in psychically and told me that the man in black had not gone over into the light and was hanging around in my office. He would be over the next day to move him on. Trying not to sound too concerned, I asked if he could come this evening rather than tomorrow, but he was busy. 'You'll be OK', he said blithely, 'just stay in your power and make the intention to be protected.' He then rang off. 'Protected from what' I thought?

As you can imagine I had a somewhat uneasy evening, constantly imagining that I heard noises and regularly looking over my shoulder. I had another restless night's sleep and woke the next morning looking forwards to Alan's visit. However, as I moved around the house and the office it felt different. The heavy atmosphere was no more and the office was back to its regular temperature. I no longer felt bothered and 'watched'. Alan arrived and went through the house, telling me that there was no spirit there; that it must have moved on during the night. 'I reckon that the energy in your office is too light because of the work that you do in here, and the spirit didn't feel comfortable there. A spirit like that prefers to be around people with dark or depressed energies. Most spirits are perfectly harmless; they're just lost or confused. However, the ones in black are the ones you have to watch out for.'

Alan told me that in all of his house clearance experiences, the vast majority of spirits leave the house and go into the light (i.e. move on in spirit to the place where they can heal) quite easily. Nearly all spirits are harmless, a few are mischievous. However, he had come upon a few which are evil or malicious. In one house, as he was trying to move on some particularly unpleasant spirits, a ceremonial sword that the house owner had hung upon the wall suddenly detached itself from its hangings and flew past Alan and embedded itself in the door behind him. I remember another friend of mine who used to work a lot with spirits (he too was a Hypnotherapist and his side-line was house clearances) telling me that once he had been picked up by unseen forces and thrown across the room in one extremely haunted house. And he weighed around 23 stones (150 kilos) at the time!

Maybe I had got away lightly, I don't know, but I was pleased to know that I was no longer sharing the house with an unwanted guest. The good thing is that Erica got better – on her next visit her mum told me that everyone around Erica was noticing big changes in her. She was more focussed, calmer and happier.

A good result all round: Final Score – Human Beings 1; Ghostly Beings 0.

Chapter 15

Healing Adult Survivors of Childhood Sex Abuse

One of the most unpleasant, and at the same time rewarding aspects of being a therapist, is helping adult survivors of childhood sex abuse. Although as a society most people seem to not want to acknowledge how widespread the sexual abuse of children is, my experience is that it is a massively under-reported problem and unfortunately it is something that I have worked with many times over the years. The reason that it is unpleasant is obvious: we have to hear our clients share their stories of the abuse and some of the things we hear are, obviously, harrowing. If you find such things too disturbing then please bypass the next two chapters and move onto Chapter 17.

Take the story of one of my clients, Mary, who was in her early 50s when she first came to see me. She was in a lot of pain and had no self-confidence. She had been brought up in a strictly religious family, all devout followers of the Salvation Army. Her parents were physically and emotionally abusive to her throughout her childhood, and when she was 12 years old her father died in front of her. Within a week a Salvation Army officer took her to their church in order, he said, to help her with her grieving. When no-one was around, he locked the door of his office, explained to her the facts of life, stripped her naked, took photos of her and raped her. He told her that God had told him to do it. This was the first time and thereafter for many years he raped her regularly, sometimes three or four times a week. She was warned not to tell anyone and he constantly told her that it was God's will that he was doing this to her. The abuse became so depraved that he was regularly buggering her, with the result that her anus and rectum was so badly damaged that she had many operations to try to repair them. When I saw her, she had no rectum left and she was in constant pain.

As you can imagine, Mary needed a lot of therapy to help her to come to terms with such horrific abuse. All sexual abuse is serious and has massive impact on the person suffering it.

I wish I could say that such clients were few and far between, but unfortunately most therapists will work regularly with people whose lives have been shattered in these ways. Although it is nearly always females who are sexually abused by males, sometimes the abuse is done by a female. One of my clients in Norway was regularly, throughout her childhood, sexually abused by her mother. She would pin her down on the floor, sometimes strangling her if she cried or moved, whilst she inserted objects into her vagina and anus and at the same time verbally abused her.

Obviously, boys are also regularly raped by men. Another of my clients was at an all-boys school, where a teacher would regularly make him stay behind after school, lock the door of a storeroom and perform sexual acts upon him.

Very occasionally a client will regress, whilst in trance, into a repressed memory of sexual abuse. This means that they recall a memory of abuse of which they had no conscious memory. This doesn't happen often as most people who have been abused remember it for all of their lives, but it happened to one of my clients who came for a smoking cessation session. Amy was in her mid-30s and had tried several times to stop smoking but she had been unable to do so. I went through my standard smoking cessation session with her and found that she was a very good trance subject. She went deeply into hypnosis and afterwards couldn't believe that she'd been in trance for more than five minutes (it was closer to fifty minutes!). She left me feeling good and confident that she was now a non-smoker. However, she called me a week later to say that she hadn't had a cigarette but she'd felt very irritable all of the time. I asked her to come back for another session and in that session, I explained to her about the possibility of her being a 'psychological smoker'. I'll explain what this means.

There are three aspects to a smoker's habit of smoking: firstly, it's a habit (always have a cup of tea or coffee, always have cigarette; always eat, always have a cigarette; always get upset, always have a cigarette etc. etc.). The vast majority of smokers build up such habits associated with smoking.

Secondly, it's an addiction. Nicotine is one of the most addictive substances known to man, and again most smokers become addicted to needing their 'fix' ten or twenty or more times a day (just like a drug addict needs to get a fix every day).

Standard hypnotherapy, in which we are using trance and post-hypnotic suggestions to re-programme the subconscious mind, is fantastic at knocking out these two aspects and allowing a person to become smoke-free quite easily.

However, the third aspect of smoking, the psychological aspect, is not widely known and I estimate connects to around ten per cent of all smokers. What this means is that a psychological smoker uses the cigarettes to subconsciously anaesthetise their inner emotional pain. EFT talks about all addictive substances (whether cigarettes, alcohol, drugs, food, chocolate etc.) being a means of softening a person's reactions to their emotional baggage. I often find that if someone comes for a smoking cessation session and afterwards they become angry or irritable, that they are almost certainly a psychological smoker. Standard hypnotherapy is usually not strong enough to deal with this.

When I explained this to Amy, she said that she knew she was carrying emotional hurts from her childhood, which was (as she said) a 'bad childhood', although she couldn't remember much of it. She realised that in order to be able to stop smoking she would need to heal some of the wounds from childhood, and she agreed to begin therapy in order to do so. I took her into hypnosis and asked her subconscious to work back into her past to uncover the significant emotional events that were causing the anger that had come through now that she was trying to stop smoking. She regressed back into several childhood memories, none of them particularly upsetting, although she did keep seeing a big, black door. Whenever she saw it, her fingers twitched involuntarily as she lay in trance. However, she couldn't relive or remember anything important, and we finished the session. I explained that sometimes the process of regression is like excavating, in that we dig down through memories until we find something of significance.

Amy returned a week or so later and told me that since our session she had felt sick whenever she thought of the black door. I guessed that this image was of great importance and once I had taken her into trance, I asked her subconscious mind to take her back into her past, to any memory that was connected to the black door. As in the previous session, she started to remember various memories from childhood.

'I'm playing in a field on my own, catching bees in a jam jar. Bees are nice.' She smiled and paused for a few seconds, before she went on: 'I'm in the street picking up stones, and now I'm playing in our back yard at home. Then I go into the passage near our house and play with my friend, Sally, and her dog. She lives next door.' Once more she paused but the smile on her face was replaced with a deep frown and she became very tense. 'I'm remembering Sally's mum screaming at me. She picks me up and she's screaming. There's blood all over my knickers. She takes me home to my mum. She puts a towel on me and takes me to hospital. I don't like it there; I just want to go home. Now I'm remembering the black door again. I'm outside the black door and I'm about 7 years old and I'm knocking on it. I remember now, it's the door to Sally's house. The door opens and her dad says that I can come in and look for her. I look for her but she's not there. Her dad won't let me go home. I want to go home. I'm wearing a white skirt. He pushes me down to the floor and holds me down. He's kneeling next to me and he takes out his penis and takes off my knickers and starts rubbing it against my thing. I can't get away; he's doing things to me. I feel sick. I can't remember anything else.'

Amy opened her eyes and came out of hypnosis understandably shocked. She had re-experienced a repressed memory from her childhood, an event of which she had no conscious awareness but which her conscious mind had suppressed because it was so traumatic. 'So that's why', she said mysteriously, and then paused for a few seconds. 'My mother had always wondered why she had come home from work one day to find that the neighbour had found me standing with my legs apart over the barbed wire fence ripping my vagina open. She had taken me to hospital but I wouldn't tell her why I had done it. It all makes so much sense now. So many things in my life are now falling into place. And that's why I've had a pain in my vagina for the past few days.'

My experience is that repressed memories are 'poisonous' memories that infect a person in so many ways without them realising. They live their lives reacting to the subconscious emotional pain that the event has locked inside them. Once they remember the hidden memory, they not only release the negative energy of the event but they are also able to integrate the fact that it happened into their lives at a conscious level and start to heal. Amy and I had more work to do to completely neutralise the negative emotions contained in that horrible event, and we did a few more sessions to fully release it. In these sessions she was able to remember more about what happened, including that the neighbour had raped her twice and performed oral sex on her. She had gone to the barbed wire fence in order to rub the 'sticky stuff' off her vagina after he had finished and threatened her not to tell anyone. In the intervening weeks between sessions she had often felt sick and upset when she thought about the incident, but in our last session she felt calm about what had happened to her and the pain in her vagina had completely gone. We did work to help her Inner Child to continue healing and she was able to start living her life much more freely than before.

It's extremely unusual for a repressed memory to appear in a hypnotherapy session, although it does very occasionally happen and once the memory has been opened up and released, the depth of the healing for the client is substantial.

These are just a small sample of such cases that I have experienced. They give a flavour of the seriousness of some of the work that we undertake as therapists. It is demanding and challenging but at the same time helping someone to overcome the wounds of childhood and to empty their emotional backpack of some of the most horrible traumas is an amazing privilege. It's said that it's never too late to enjoy a happy childhood.

Chapter 16

The Horrors of a Satanic Paedophile Ring

Much like Amy in the last chapter, Sarah came to me not realising that her subconscious was holding onto a mass of repressed memories. The way in which they came out is fascinating, even though the nature of the memories is highly disturbing. She was in her early 40s and had been suffering from ME (Myalgic Encephalomyelitis), a form of Chronic Fatigue Syndrome, for over five years. As well as feeling constantly exhausted, there were times when she felt so ill that she could only speak and think with difficulty and she was unable to express herself. She couldn't work (having previously had a career in business) and spent a lot of the time in bed. The one bright thing in her life was her husband Pete, who she described as her 'rock'. Pete sat in on all of her therapy sessions with me, observing the regression process, and I'm so pleased that he did as he is able to verify that at no stage did I lead or implant any leading suggestions into Sarah, but that everything that happened in our sessions (and also after our sessions) was presented by her subconscious in its own incredible way.

In answer to my questions about traumas in her life, Sarah listed a few, including a childhood which was spoilt by her father. She said that he was 'a real arse' and that he had suppressed her and her sister and their mother by being constantly controlling and verbally aggressive. Her mother was scared of him and never challenged him or his behaviour. As a result Sarah felt let down by her mother, who had never protected her from his psychopathic actions.

These traumas in themselves could be enough to have caused her ME, but once she went into trance and her subconscious had created an Ideo-Motor Response, her finger signalled that the emotional causes of her illness were not only the traumas in this present lifetime but also in several past lives as well as the lives of some of her ancestors. I was wondering if we would spend time regressing into significant emotional events from this lifetime in our first session, but her subconscious (which usually knows the best healing process, and definitely did in Sarah's case) took us into the first of the past lives. She went straight into a terrifying death experience, and as she gasped out her words to tell me what she was seeing she was crying throughout the experience:

I feel really hot and I can smell burning. I'm in a clearing in a wood and I'm standing with my hands tied behind my back to a stake. I'm a young woman and my head is tied too with a rope around my forehead. I'm being burnt at the stake. I don't want to die. I can't get away; I'm frightened. I can see someone with a flaming torch; it's going to burn my long hair. My feet are bare and I'm wearing my wedding dress. My husband's made me wear it; he's watching; he wants me dead. He wants this.

With these words Sarah began to sob loudly and writhe around in the chair, as if trying to get away from the flames. Her words came out in short, sharp gasps.

I've done something wrong but I don't know what I've done wrong. I gave a poor man some apples and spoke to him. I was just being kind. His family have made him do this because I've shamed the family. He's had to do this for his family's name. He's staring into my eyes and he won't drop his gaze. I was doing things for the poor and they didn't like it. They made him do this — it's done in secret, that's why I've been taken away into the woods. They don't understand me. Some of their faces are looking on in shock and horror. My husband just holds my gaze. I loved him so much.

With these words Sarah slowly began to calm down and after a while her crying stopped and she relaxed. Eventually she spoke quietly: *'I think I'm dead now; I feel cool and calm. I'm at peace and feeling light'*. I gave Sarah time to relax again and go into a deeper trance and I asked her if anyone in that life has been around her in this lifetime. Immediately she replied that her husband in the past life is her father in this present life. As she said this she began to shiver and breathe quickly; her subconscious had taken her into another past life. I asked her to tell me what she was seeing. Her words came with a stutter, as if she was freezing:

> *I'm a little girl, about 8 or 9 years old; I'm outside and I'm crouched down in a doorway. I'm really cold. We're huddled together; my mum and baby brother and me. I'm wearing rags and I'm dirty. It's so cold. My brother is so small. People go by; horses and carts go by. My left arm is broken. A horrible man has come; he smells horrible of drink and he's dirty. Oh, he smells! He wants my mum — he's going to take her.* Sarah became agitated and she started to cry. *He's not my dad. I'm holding onto her but he's hitting me and he breaks my arm. He's trying to take her away. I can't move, I have to be quiet. I stay with my brother Joe and rock him so he stops crying. He takes mum across the street. She doesn't come back to us but later I see her in the doorway with her head hanging and her eyes open. That's when we huddle up to her; we want her to wake up. I've died now but I can't move on as I'm waiting for my brother. He comes and so it's OK to leave mum now and go to the light. I feel calm and at peace and happy with Joe.*

I asked her if she recognised the man from that life and she began to cry as she said that it was her father in this life. The session was over and when she came out of trance Sarah was tired but relieved, as well as very surprised at what had come through in the past lifetimes. She was pleased that we had begun the journey of working on the energetic causes of her ME, and when she returned with Pete a couple of weeks later, she told me that she felt lighter as a result of the past lives we had worked through, especially with regards to her dad. She now felt that she'd let go of a feeling of responsibility that she'd always had towards him, and she no longer felt that she had to look for his approval. Although she was still fatigued most of the time, she felt changes were happening inside her.

Once she was into trance in this session she went into another past life, this time as a young soldier in the trenches in WWI. Her arms moved in front of her, as if she was holding a rifle. She whispered the words to me as I asked her to share with me what she was experiencing:

> *It's dark and I'm keeping quiet. My heart's racing. I don't know what's going to happen. My back's against the trench and I think I'm the only one alive. The others are dead in the trench. We've been blown up. My legs have gone. I see my friend to my left slumped over. We would smoke and play cards together and he asks me to give his family a letter if he dies; I can't do that now. Some Germans are coming over the top of the trench; they're all laughing. I'm praying to God. They've put my eyes out. One of them just stands there laughing and he orders his men to do it.* Sarah was shifting around in the chair as if trying to get away. Her speech became slurred: *They cut my tongue out and take my insides out. They cut my hands off — I was praying. I can't hear properly because of the bomb blast. They leave me. I'm still alive. One of them comes and I can feel that he's sorry. He shoots me in the head. I feel better now; calm, and I can see lots of nice colours.*

Sarah slumped down in the chair and was still. Then she became emotional as she said:

The laughing German who made them do it is my father.

The association of her father ordering her to be brutalised in that life triggered her subconscious to take her into another experience, but this time she had moved not into another previous life but into an ancestor's life. Surprisingly, she moved into the life of her father:

> *I'm a little boy, around* 3 *or* 4 *and I'm being beaten and it hurts. I'm my dad when he's tiny. My dad* (i.e. Sarah's grandfather) *is hitting me with a piece of wood and I'm on the floor. I'm being sick and I've wet myself. My brother's just laughing. My mum's not stopping it. I probably got the blame for my brother; he never gets in trouble. I'm cowering on the floor and then my dad goes out. I don't even get a hug from my mum and I have to sort myself out. I cuddle my teddy bear. I don't want to be there as I always get picked on.*

Sarah was silent for a couple of minutes and then she stopped crying and she became calm. She told me that the images had gone which signalled the end of the regression experience so I brought her back to full awareness. She was amazed that she had regressed into her father's childhood and that she had felt like she was actually in *his* body as a small child, seeing and feeling *his* father (her grandfather) beating him. As I said earlier on in this book, in regression sessions we are releasing the locked-in emotions and energies from three different areas: from this present life, from our previous lives, and from the traumas that we inherit from ancestors in our bloodline (parents, grandparents, great-grandparents, great-great-grandparents etc. etc.). Usually when we relive ancestral trauma in this way we are simply releasing the emotions and energies that are in our emotional pressure cooker; sometimes though as a result of this we gain a greater understanding of our ancestor and why they have been the way they are throughout their life. This reframe can create a healing between the ancestor (if they are still alive) and the client. Often, as in Sarah's case, she re-lived her father being physically abused in childhood and came to realise that one reason why her father had been behaving so badly all of her life is because he was abused in his. This realisation that her father had simply been reacting to his own inner pain was a first step towards being open to the possibility of forgiving him for damaging her so much throughout her life.

At the start of her next session Sarah told me that she had talked with her dad about her experience in regression of being beaten by his father and he confirmed that this did happen as she described it. She was anxious about what was to come in this new session as she felt it would contain some unpleasant information, but she was happy to go into hypnosis to see what her subconscious wanted her to work on. Within a few minutes she started to wring her hands together and her face looked severe and pained. I asked her to describe what she was experiencing:

> *My heart's pounding; I think I'm in a damp cell, chained to a wall. It's quiet and dark but there are rats running around. I'm tired, thin and hungry. I'm a Jew in a prison camp. I'm a scientist, a Professor. It's hard to breathe and I'm cold. I haven't got my glasses. I feel so sad; I've done something I know will kill lots of people. I didn't know that was how it was going to be used. It's a liquid that we made to gas the Jews. I can hear shooting — a firing squad outside. I know some of the people I've been working with have been shot and I feel so ashamed about what my work has done. I'm just wasting away and I want to die. I see images of children running scared in my memory. They're being split up from their parents and then measured with a stick. If they're under it they go one way; if taller they go the other. Lots of the boys have just shorts and a*

vest on and no shoes. I'm given some info about the children — how many, what size. I have a formula. I put numbers into the formula and work out the amounts needed. I'm writing it down — all the different amounts of substances and chemicals to create the liquid gas. I know I'm doing it.

Throughout all of this Sarah was struggling to hold back the tears, but finally she started to cry softly as she continued:

It's the solution. It's all so matter of fact; *we all have no choice. We know what we're doing but we can do nothing about it. I start writing a formula. I have my head in my hands on my bench; it's eating me away. When they come for me, I can't do it anymore. They make me write out the formula. It's hard to breathe. I'm in a room with a light on the desk. I have to say "Mein Fuhrer".* (As she said this her arm went up into the air into a Nazi salute.) *They hit me in the stomach. I'm being punched and beaten and forced to write the formula. There's blood on my paper where I have to write the formula. I'm in my shorts and vest, just like the boys being measured. I can't write it; I can't leave it to them. I'm so thirsty. Someone else walks in, an older man, but I can't stand up so they punch me to make me stand up. I've made my decision — I'll die. They can kill me but I can't let any more children die. They can do whatever they want to me; I've already killed so many. I can't give them the formula. I'm paraded around the lab. I'm half dead, covered in blood and my face is unrecognisable. My leg and arm are broken. I was dragged around the lab and then taken here. I can't move. Someone else is in this room, like me he's slumped against the wall. He's bloodied and his face is misshapen. Why can't I die? Please God, save me. In the beginning we didn't know — we thought we were going to be pioneers to create something great and amazing to save lives. We were hired as a special elite. We were so excited and proud to be part of this special unit. We all worked so hard. They said to us that there is a race and we had to work quickly. So we did. But then we knew. I'm so sorry. We did a terrible thing and I can't forgive myself. I have to punish myself somehow for this.*

Eventually Sarah stopped crying as she died and passed into spirit and then was silent for a time before she came out of trance. She told me that she understood now why she had never allowed herself to have children in this present lifetime, and how she'd punished herself throughout this life in different ways. She said that her current illness was her final punishment. We talked about the past life and although she was sombre when we finished the session, she felt calm when she left.

In our next few sessions Sarah regressed into her mother's life and experienced (as her mother) being sexually abused by her mother's father (in other words Sarah's grandfather) in her childhood and teens. This was obviously very upsetting for Sarah and was not something that she knew anything about. She asked her mother if the abuse had actually occurred and her mum confirmed that it had, although she didn't want to talk about it as she'd never told anyone before and had locked it inside her all of her life.

We spent the next few months regressing back into events in Sarah's present life that had traumatised her, including releasing the remnants of meningitis in her energy field which she had caught in her 20s. We also had one more past life to release in which she was in Atlantis at the time that it was overwhelmed by water and lost beneath the seas. She felt like she was with others in a position of authority in Atlantis and that they were trying to keep control against greed and corruption but that they failed and Atlantis was destroyed.

As a result of our therapy sessions Sarah's health got better and better. She not only felt emotionally calmer, happier and much more balanced than she ever had felt before, the ME went into remission and her natural energy returned. She was able to start to live a normal life again and I honestly believed that we had done everything in our sessions to get her back to full health again and that there was nothing else to do. When she left my office after our final session, I didn't think I would ever see her or Pete again. How wrong I was!

Two years later Sarah called me on the phone sounding troubled. Although she was still feeling healthy and the ME had not returned, she said that she had started getting memories of childhood sex abuse popping up into her mind from time to time. She couldn't make sense of the memories as she couldn't see them clearly but she thought that they involved her maternal grandpa and her grandmother (who she called 'nana'). We talked for a while and I expressed doubt that the memories could be real. We had done so much regression work two years earlier that I would have expected that if she had been sexually abused in childhood such memories would have appeared at some stage during our sessions. However, I agreed that we could investigate further and Sarah and Pete came to my office a few days later. We talked about the possibility that she had been sexually abused but she had no conscious memories of any such incidents, and once more I expressed doubts that she had been abused. I shared with her the theory that sometimes people think that they have been abused, possibly because they read or hear about childhood sex abuse and they start to wonder if such a thing happened to them. The more they dwell on such a possibility the more likely it is that they imagine that they have been abused and they create false memories of being abused. Although for most people it is difficult to create such false memories, some people are able to do so.

I wanted to be careful that I didn't lead Sarah into any such false memories, so once she was in hypnosis I simply asked her to go back into her childhood in order to remember any memories from childhood that her subconscious wanted her to revisit.

Within seconds she was reliving a memory of her grandpa and nana playing doctors and nurses with her when she was a little girl, around 3 years old. She was naked, her legs and arms were tied down and they were touching her and putting things into her vagina and warning her not to tell anyone about it. Grandpa then penetrated her with his penis whilst nana watched, put his penis into her mouth and then ejaculated onto her stomach. Finally he urinated on her.

As she was describing this to me, at times Sarah was talking like a little girl, giving details of what was happening in a childlike way, as if she was in the body of a 3-year-old girl as these awful things happened to her. I brought Sarah out of trance and although she was understandably shocked at what she'd experienced, she also said that she felt a strange feeling of 'knowing' that the memory was real. She knew that her relationship with her grandparents had always been weird, and that she had spent a lot of time at their house throughout her childhood. I wasn't convinced though that the memory Sarah had described was real, although I have to say that the fact that she had experienced the memory of abuse so vividly and was so 'associated' (in other words in the body rather than describing the scene and the events from a distance in a 'disassociated' state) and talking like a child at times suggested that it was a real incident. We agreed to do more regressions in order to see if we could make sense of things.

This was the start of a process in which, over many hypnotherapy sessions, Sarah regressed back into childhood and relived many events of sexual abuse and ritualistic satanic abuse at the hands of her grandpa and nana. When I started to write this chapter I was intending to write in detail about what her abusers had done to her, but once I reread the notes that I made in the therapy sessions I realised that the graphic nature of the abuse was so unpleasant and disgusting that it would alter the whole tone of this book and perhaps be so abhorrent for a general reader that they may not want to read on. So, instead of writing Sarah's memories and sharing her words from the regressions, in which she re-experienced them in an associated state and talked like a child, I have decided to summarise the nature of the abuse without all of the lurid details. This may be less graphic, but is still shocking.

The experiences of sexual abuse started when Sarah was around 3 and continued throughout her childhood into her early teens. The initial experiences were almost in the nature of 'grooming' the little girl into getting used to being touched and handled sexually. These incidents took place at the grandparents' house and in these the grandparents would turn the abuse into games, even though they often consisted of rape and oral sex. Sometimes Sarah was tied down and as well as being molested she was forced to watch her grandparents having oral sex and penetrative sex. Little Sarah was consistently warned not to tell anyone, especially not her parents. These threats were done in a variety of ways, sometimes to scare her ('you're a bad girl and bad things will happen to you if you tell'), sometimes to confuse her ('no-one will ever believe you') and sometimes to threaten her ('grandpa will be angry and will hurt you').

After a while a new tactic was introduced, that of drugging Sarah before the abuse took place. This was done by getting her to drink something which had a drug in it. Sarah wasn't completely knocked out by the drug but she was woozy and unable to control her body or fight off her abusers. When she was a little older (maybe 7 or 8) her grandparents started to take her to Satanic rituals in which she was tied down and groups of men would molest her. Sometimes they would be wearing cloaks and chanting as they took turns to rape her; other times they would be naked and contorting themselves around her. Often there would be other children around; some of them would be abused too whilst some would be there in order to groom them and prepare them for future ceremonies in which they would be abused. One ritual which was particularly terrifying for the young Sarah was when they used a knife (probably a stage knife) to pretend to cut her and carve symbols on her naked body. The knife would leave a trail of blood on her skin which they would then lick off her. It appeared that her grandparents were either the organisers of this satanic coven or were high up in the hierarchy.

An especially horrible piece of emotional abuse that went along with these horrific acts was her grandparents telling the young Sarah that her parents were not actually her parents, but that they (the grandparents) were her real parents. That's why her parents didn't love her, but they (the grandparents) did.

This brief description of the evils that were perpetrated upon her only give a flavour of the hideous nature of the emotional, physical and sexual abuse that took place. As you can imagine, it was harrowing for me and Sarah's husband Pete to spend each session listening to Sarah describe these traumas from her childhood, and of course even more harrowing for her to bring each memory out into the open. Over time, though, Sarah felt more and more released from these terrible events and she began to feel lighter and happier and freer. The whole aim of the regression process was to release the traumas which had been hidden in her subconscious for so long and to heal her of the damage that these events had done to her physically, mentally, emotionally and even spiritually. It was as though, over time, we had gone into many rooms in her mind which had been locked for years and which contained darkness and pain. We had let the light into those rooms and released the darkness before making sure that those rooms only contained light and beauty. I often talk about the breathtaking wisdom that the subconscious has and the wondrous ability that it has in order to heal, and this was shown in the way that her subconscious controlled her healing process. It's as though it knew that when we first worked together a couple of years earlier that Sarah was not ready to be shown the sexual abuse in her childhood. But once we had worked on and let go of the other significant emotional events from the past and once she had a couple of years to process those sessions and to start to stabilise mentally and emotionally, her subconscious knew that she was stronger and it was now safe for her to be shown the sexual abuse memories. For me, that is a phenomenal wisdom.

Since our sessions together Sarah has continued to heal, to grow spiritually and to blossom as a human being. After our final session together Sarah wrote to me to thank me and to tell me how she felt. Her words carry much beauty and an energy of wellbeing that they bounce off the page:

Steve, I believe a miracle occurred. As a child, to survive the abuse I split off so many parts of myself — hundreds I'm sure — and the miracle is that they're back and in that process brought light and love and possibility into my life that I never knew was possible. I feel whole and complete but bigger somehow and the power within me is so new. I am healing myself. I keep saying it's me, it's me, it's me who experienced those horrors and it's me sat here smiling. With your love you have helped this miracle to happen, a true miracle of healing, thank you from all of me.

Chapter 17

There's Nothing Wrong with Me. Oh, There Is...

'See the happy moron, he doesn't give a damn.
I wish I was a moron; my God, perhaps I am!'
— Anon

I'm sometimes asked if I have ever had therapy myself, and people are often surprised to find that I have, as if they think that as a therapist, I must be perfect in all ways and immune to the stresses of life. I still have regular therapy sessions as I want to let go of 'stuff' that is stopping me from living my life freely, although when I first began my career I didn't think in this way. Like many therapists I thought that I didn't have issues but only my clients did; which of course was a foolish way of thinking, because we all have baggage of some sort. John Bradshaw, the father of Inner Child therapy, has said that only 4% of people are truly functional, which means that 96% of us are screwed up in some way! Personally, I think that less than 1% of people are truly functional, and I've met very few totally balanced people during the course of my life who would be in that 1% (one who springs to mind is a Tibetan lama who I met during a retreat I attended at a Tibetan monastery in Scotland).

So my first experience of having therapy was something of a dramatic initiation into the world of trance. It was an experience that changed my life and made me a better human being and a better therapist. This took place about 6 months after I'd done my initial hypnotherapy training and started working with clients in my therapy practice. I began to realise that I didn't know enough to work totally effectively with clients so I decided to re-train and attend a week-long hypnotherapy training course run by Wilf Proudfoot, who subsequently became my mentor until his death in 2013.

I'd always been the class joker at school, so as I sat on the course in a group of around 40 people, I reverted to type and sometimes would throw in funny comments to amuse the group. Wilf was at the front of the group, demonstrating therapy techniques by working with members of the group on different issues. On the second day of the course I said something which got a laugh but Wilf, who was sitting at the front heard me and said 'Steve, that's the second time you've said something about fathers. Come up here.'

'Eh?' was my shocked response.

'Yes, come up here, I think there's something we can work on for you.'

'Oh shit', I thought, 'I've done it now.' With my heart in my mouth I went to the front of the class and sat next to Wilf, with everyone looking at me expectantly. I suddenly felt very nervous. I'd watched Wilf working like this with group members and seen some people become quite emotional when they worked on their issues. I wondered just what was going to come up for me; I hoped I wouldn't be embarrassed.

'OK', Wilf said gently, 'tell me a little about your relationship with your dad.'

Somewhat reluctantly, as I've always been a private person and talking about myself in front of so many people made me feel quite vulnerable and exposed, I told Wilf that I never felt that my dad was there for me in childhood as he was always working and trying to create an important life for himself.

I should say that this is a common issue, felt by many people. The wonderful pioneer of family therapy, Virginia Satir, called such issues 'Universalisms'. Just as an aside, for those who know of NLP, Virginia was one of the three pioneering therapists that were analysed by the creators of NLP to create the models and systems that later grew into Neuro-linguistic Programming.

Wilf Proudfoot and Virginia Satir were close friends in the latter years of her life and she was regularly referred to by Wilf during his training courses. I often feel the influence of that legacy in my work as a therapist.

A second great therapist modelled by the NLP creators was Fritz Perls, who created Gestalt Therapy. It was at this stage in my session that Wilf moved into using Gestalt Therapy with me. As he sat at the side of me, he pulled up an empty chair and placed it in front of me. 'Put your dad in that chair and tell him what you want to tell him about your childhood', he said softly. What follows here is a shortened version of my therapy session but it'll give you an idea of the process.

Feeling a bit confused I imagined my dad sitting looking at me and I spoke out loud to my imaginary dad telling him how I thought he hadn't been there for me. Falteringly, as I was very conscious of many pairs of eyes in the room watching me expectantly, I said 'Dad, I want to tell you that you didn't spend time with me as a child. I wanted some attention from you; I wanted you to play football with me and play with me. I resent that you didn't, that you were always working and you had no time for me.'

Wilf then asked me to swap chairs and become my dad. I sat in my dad's chair and looked at my empty chair and imagined I was my dad talking to me in that empty chair. 'You've heard what Steve has to say dad, how do you respond?' Wilf said. I then spoke as if I was my dad answering the things I had just said to him:

'You have to see it from my point of view; I had nothing as a child, we were very poor and I always wanted the best for you so you could have the things I never had as a child.'

When I had finished speaking, Wilf had me sit back in my chair and reply to my imaginary dad in his chair, responding to what he (enacted by me, of course) had just said. This process went on for some time, with me swapping chairs and having a dialogue with my imaginary dad and me. Throughout the whole time I was very tense, my hands clasped tightly together and my body language betraying the feelings I was subconsciously feeling. I could feel myself getting more and more uptight as the forgotten emotions of childhood started to be opened up. I continued to respond to my imaginary dad:

'You've always seen things wrongly; your dominating factor has been to achieve things at the expense of love. I resent that.' I swapped chairs and became my dad, and I could feel myself becoming more and more chewed up inside.

'I don't understand you; I needed to be someone, to have money. I wanted to achieve things for myself that would bring the best for you. I didn't want you to grow up in the poverty that I lived through as a child.'

Wilf sat me back in my chair and said 'Try this. Look at your dad and say "I love you"'. After a long pause, with emotion in my voice, I quietly said 'dad, I love you'.

I swapped chairs again and Wilf said to me as my dad 'Dad, how do you feel as Steve says that he loves you? How do you reply to him?'

I closed my eyes and said 'I feel a real desire for love. I say to Steve, I love you too and have always loved you. But you know my way is to show love without showing love.' I opened my eyes and looked across at the imaginary Steve. 'You don't know what it's like to grow up in poverty. My father died when I was young so I've had no role model to follow as a parent. I had to do the best for myself.'

I swapped chairs again and responded vehemently to my dad: 'I feel angry, you're fooling yourself, you can't see anything from anyone else's point of view.' Wilf asked me what my anger was telling me and suddenly the direction of the session changed as in my anger I said loudly 'I want you to let me live the life I want to live. I want to be my own person, not domineered by you. I want to tell you that it won't work anymore, I'm not going to be controlled anymore.'

Wilf asked me how I was feeling, and I said that I felt relief. I'd got something off my chest that was hiding underneath the layers of stuff from my childhood. Subconscious tension that I'd always felt but never verbalised was out in the open. Wilf asked me to become my dad again, in his chair, and said 'Dad, you've heard Steve say that he's not going to let you domineer him anymore. What do you have to say to him?' As my dad, I felt myself soften and smile as I replied: 'I respect you for that. You're a Clever Dick though! I'll always be there for you if you need me.'

It seemed that we'd achieved a resolution between my imaginary dad and me, Wilf asked me how I felt. He'd been observing me closely throughout the session and could see how uncomfortable I was. 'I feel very emotional', I said. 'It's like there's a knot of tightness in my chest.'

My head was down, my hands were clasping tightly together and my jaw felt locked. 'Then let yourself feel it', Wilf said, 'it's okay to feel it.'

'I can't', I said, 'in front of all these people.'

'Just look at all these people', Wilf replied, and he made me look around the half circle of therapists in the room watching my session. I did so, and I could see in most people's eyes sympathy and I all could feel coming to me from the group was love. Some of them were quietly crying, as their childhood issues of rejection were being triggered too. 'It's such a shame that men find it hard to cry', said Wilf 'but it's so important that we allow ourselves to feel emotions. I did some group work like this myself some years ago and a lot of emotion came through for me. I've seen Churchill cry several times' (Wilf was a former Member of Parliament). 'Close your eyes Steve and stay with those feelings.'

I could feel a wave of grief starting to churn around in my chest. It got stronger and stronger until I could hold it in no longer. Wilf put his hand on my shoulder reassuringly and suddenly I started to weep uncontrollably. Wilf pulled me towards him and held me in his arms, stroking my back and shoulders quietly saying 'feel the emotion and let it go, it's OK to feel the feelings'.

I sat sobbing whilst he hugged me for some time before the emotions subsided. All the time Wilf just held me and spoke gently to me that it's fine to allow oneself to feel and release such a lot of grief. After a while the tears ceased to flow and I breathed a big sigh of relief. I sat upright again and Wilf asked me how I felt. 'Released' was the word I used.

I was able to breathe freely again and the knot of emotional pain in my chest had gone. I felt calmer and more at ease; when I thought of my dad and the issue of feeling abandoned that I had been working on I wasn't triggered anymore. As well as this, a part of my mind had reframed the conflict I had been feeling towards him so I was able to understand his reasons for having to spend less time with the family when I was growing up. Something had shifted inside me and I felt inner peace.

As I wrote at the start of this chapter, this therapy session changed my life. Not only did I release emotions that had been locked inside of me since childhood that were unconsciously affecting me, but I also learnt that it's OK for men to cry and to feel their feelings. I felt freer inside myself than I'd ever felt and I was able to let go of the repressed anger I'd held towards my dad since childhood. I think that on that day I became a bigger person and I learnt as a therapist that it is OK to allow my clients to cry and to feel their emotions. I'll always be grateful to Wilf Proudfoot for pulling me out from the class that day and making me work on my 'stuff'. I also owe him so much for the influence he had upon my subsequent career.

Chapter 18

Working on the Root Causes of Phobias

Phobias are always interesting things to work with. I usually say that there are 'degrees' of phobias, which means that a person suffering from one can either have a light phobic reaction, a medium reaction or a severe reaction. For example, someone who has light state of agoraphobia (a fear of open spaces) will feel uncomfortable being outside in nature or in a large shopping centre. Someone with a medium state of agoraphobia will not feel good when they are away from home or in a street a short distance away from their home. Someone with a severe state of agoraphobia will rarely leave their house. Twenty years ago I worked with a lady who was so severely agoraphobic that she hadn't stepped outside of her front door for several years. The mere thought of actually doing so would make her feel very panicky. Many people with light to medium phobias are able to live their lives relatively normally; a person with a severe phobia will find that it affects their life and stops them from living their life freely, and they have to live each day within the confines set by their fear.

Every phobia has a long name (e.g. claustrophobia, which is a fear of enclosed spaces), and there are phobias for just about everything on the planet. Hypnotherapists are often called to treat many common phobias, such as spiders, mice, vomit (emetophobia), snakes, clowns, heights, social situations, and birds; as well as uncommon phobias such as thunder and lightning, beards, cheese, belly buttons, writing in public, the colour yellow, the number four, leaves, books and crossing roads, to name just a few. Like I said, there are phobias for virtually everything. I heard of a lady in the UK a few years ago who had a phobia of the holes in the middle of donuts!

Whenever she saw a donut, she would go to pieces; watching an episode of The Simpsons must have been excruciating for her. There is even a phobia of having peanut butter stuck to the roof of your mouth (arachibutyrophobia if you must know).

Sometimes phobias can be released or neutralised very quickly (there are several Neuro-Linguistic Programming techniques which can often work in minutes), but some phobias are very tough to work with and can take several sessions to clear. Although we can learn a phobia of spiders by regularly being exposed in childhood, say, to a parent who becomes terrified and screams when they see a spider, the vast majority of phobias are caused by locked-in feelings and emotions from past traumas.

A good example of this is when I worked with Vicky, a retired lady who had suffered from a phobia of dogs for all of her life. She told me that she couldn't remember anything that had ever happened to start the phobia; she had always been terrified of dogs as long as she could remember. She was so scared that she rarely went out of her house, and on the rare occasions when she plucked up courage to go shopping or into a town centre, she had to have several people with her (all walking around her) in case she saw a dog. If she saw a dog she would scream and shake and have a panic attack. This was obviously a severe phobia as it stopped her from living her life freely. I mentioned to her that as part of the treatment protocol I might give her a hypnosis relaxation recording to play at home, in which she would imagine herself relaxing in a beautiful place in nature, but she told me that she would 'flip out' if she played it as she always associated open spaces with dogs. This truly was a severe phobia.

She wanted to become free of the fear of dogs as she was about to visit her daughter in the USA. She told me that her daughter had a big dog and when Vicky visited in the past the dog had had to be put into kennels. She felt this was unfair to both the dog and her daughter's family.

When she went into trance, I asked her subconscious to take her back to the root cause of the phobia, and after a couple of minutes I saw a quizzical look on her face and her eyelids started to flicker (a sign that she was visualising something). I asked her to tell me what she was seeing and she told me that she was remembering being 2 years old and her mum was strapping her into a buggy to go for a walk. She then told me that she was being pushed in the buggy by her mum to the park, where mum wheeled her to the duck pond to watch the ducks. Mum then walked off to speak to a friend. She felt comfortable watching the ducks and birds on the water. She was smiling and breathing in a relaxed way for a while, and then suddenly her whole demeanour changed in an instant. Her face looked troubled, her body went as stiff as a board and her breathing started to race. She pulled her head over to one side, as if trying to get away from something. I asked her to tell me what she was seeing. She spoke through gritted teeth:

'A dog. A dog's here and it's sniffing me. It's sniffing me!'

She started to cry and suddenly her right arm came up and hit the imaginary dog, as if she was trying to bat it away. Immediately she let out an enormous scream and she held on to her right cheek with her hands. Her legs were kicking in the chair and she threw herself from side to side, all the time yelling and screaming and sobbing. 'It's bitten me. It bit me on my cheek' she yelled between gasps. 'Mummy, mummy, mummy' she cried out several times, before finally subsiding into painful whimpers, as if she was remembering being comforted in her mother's arms.

Once we had fully released the fear and pain from the memory, we did some Inner Child therapy to make sure that her 2-year-old self felt calm and safe and then I brought Vicky out of trance. She was amazed at how vivid the experience had been, even though she was re-living a forgotten memory from more than 50 years earlier. She told me that having re-experienced it she knew that the memory was real. As she was looking at the ducks in the park, a large dog had come over to sniff her. It kept putting its nose into her face and she smacked it to make it go away; the dog bit her on the cheek and she was terrified. What was worse was that she was strapped into the buggy so she was trapped and couldn't get away.

In the weeks after, as she prepared for her holiday in the States, she was able to stroke a dog for the first time in her life (what's more, it was a Great Dane!) and she felt more confident in herself. She was walking more instead of driving everywhere; the phobia was gone.

A couple of months after our session there was a knock at my office door, and there was Vicky with several holiday photos, showing her sitting next to her daughter's dog and also sitting with the dog in the car. I still have the photos as a memento of a fascinating case.

***

Another interesting case was that of Paul, a business owner who had a phobia of needles and blood (as well as anything to do with hospitals). He had broken his leg and was very stressed about being treated for it, especially in terms of having injections. He was a strong man in many ways, but he simply went to pieces whenever he had to have an injection. He hobbled into my office on crutches with his leg in a plaster cast, and once we had talked about his fears, I guided him into hypnosis. Once in trance I asked his subconscious to create an IMR signal and his whole right hand floated up into the air, as if it were a helium-filled balloon. His subconscious then indicated that the causes of his phobia of needles and blood were in two previous lives, and we worked in both of them in one session. He went quickly into the first past life, and with his eyes closed he began to tell me what he was seeing:

> *It's medieval times and I'm a man with lots of people at a banquet. There's lots of noise, laughter and music. People are*

drinking and enjoying themselves. It feels good to be there; some people are dancing. At first Paul seemed amused by what he was experiencing, but suddenly he became serious and his body jerked and went into a spasm as he hissed:

There's a fight; there's lots of fighting. I get stabbed in the stomach. I've fallen to the floor. I'm crying as I lay on the floor; I don't want to die. I die slowly. I don't want to leave my wife.

After a few minutes of tense breathing Paul finally relaxed as he experienced leaving his body and moving into Spirit. We went back through the stabbing and death several times in order to fully release the tensions and negative emotions, and once he was able to relive it without any feelings I moved him into the next past life. In this one he was a gangster in Chicago:

It's night-time and I'm riding on the running board of a big, black car. I'm holding a machine gun as we drive down a dark street. I'm firing the gun; shooting at the windows of a large building. There's glass falling and shattering everywhere. A large piece of it falls and gets stuck in my arm and I'm bleeding real badly. I feel like I'm going to pass out. I fall off the car but it just drives off and leaves me in the gutter bleeding. I'm laid in a pool of blood, dying.

Throughout this Paul was squirming in the chair, his face was white and he felt sick as he remembered the feelings of blood pouring out of his body as he died. Once he had died and felt calm, we went through it again a few times so he could fully let go of the trauma, and then I brought him back out of trance. He felt very relaxed and free inside. A couple of days later he had an injection at the hospital and he had no problems at all.

***

By way of contrast, another example of a client with a phobia of needles is the case of Alex, a 40-year-old nurse who had left her job in a local hospital to work in the national blood transfusion service. She'd always felt anxious around syringes but her new job of taking blood all day triggered a fear of injecting people that was causing her constant stress. She felt anxious before she got to work each day and being at work was a struggle as she had to expend a lot of energy pushing down her fears so that no-one could see that she was uptight. Can you imagine how it must feel to be a nurse with a phobia of injecting people, who has to do blood transfusions all day?

We discovered that there were traumas in several former lives as well as in one of her ancestors' lives that was at the heart of the phobia. The first past life contained a theme that has featured in many of my client's previous lives over the years (which I'll be covering in more depth later), that of being persecuted and killed for being a witch:

> *I'm outdoors and it's daytime; I'm a woman in my mid-20s. I'm standing alone in the woods; I'm frightened. Someone's told me that they're coming after me. I go to my house; there are different plants and things laid out on a long table. There are lots of pungent smells. I'm pouring from a big jug into a smaller jug and I give it to an old man who's come to see me. His joints hurt. Someone else comes with a baby but it's dead and I can't help them; I feel sad.*

Alex was quiet for a minute or so before she became tense. I asked her what was happening and she replied with fear in her voice:

> *I'm sat at the table looking at the fire. I'm alone. I'm scared because I can see things before they happen. I can hear a lot of noise — men on horseback. They've come for taxes but people can't pay. One of the cottages in the village is burning. There's*

a big man standing in the doorway, he comes in and turns the table upside down. He's calling me a witch. I feel frightened but I'm not going to let him see that. He's one of the local lords and he killed my father for poaching on the land. He hits me and he's dragging me by my hair. He twists my left arm and it hurts; I think he's broken it. He kicks me in the ribs and my lip's bleeding. He's got his hand around my throat, pushing me against the wall. I hate him. I feel a dagger in my hand, from the belt at my side — I use it to cut things for the potions. I push the knife into his stomach and feel his blood on my hands. I hate him.

Again Alex paused and her breathing began to slow down. She started to cry softly as she continued:

I'm in a cold, stone-walled dungeon. I killed him. I'm not as frightened now as I know I'm going to die. I'm sad. They hang me. I feel peace now, I'm not there anymore and I'm floating into the light. I feel at peace.

Alex breathed a sigh of relief and softened into the chair. She was calm for a short time and then she moved into another life and her body became tense again. As her hands clenched into fists she began to speak:

I'm outdoors on a battlefield; there's lots of noise — explosions and people crying out in pain. I'm in a trench in the First World War and I'm a young man, about 18 *years old. I'm frightened and cold, there's lots of blood and people laid out all around me shouting for medics. There's been no let-up of firing at each other. I feel* 50, *not* 18, *and I'm thinking about the pointlessness of it all. I'm sitting in the trench now with my hands around a metal cup; it's supposed to be tea but it's more like cloudy water, though at least it's warming my hands.*

I've seen a lot of pointless action and lost a lot of my friends. We all started out together and everyone was waving as we were leaving — "we're gonna win this war". Look at us now. I'm from Leicester but I seem to have been in this muddy field for a long time. It doesn't turn my stomach anymore seeing people blown up.

Now that she'd set the scene, I asked her to move to the significant event that connected to the phobia in this lifetime. She winced and her body suddenly jerked upwards:

A bayonet going right through me; there's pain right through my back and blood all over my hands. There's no-one to call for help as the rest of 'em are dead. I don't want to die in this God-forsaken place. I'm laid on my back looking up at the night sky and the stars — I feel the stars are coming down towards me; I think I'm getting delirious. She started to shake and shiver. *I'm getting very cold. I think about putting a gun to my head, it'll make it quicker. Is that being a coward? I'm only* 18 *and I was going to do so much — now I won't be doing anything. I see nothing now, I'm light and floating. I'm looking down on my body, it's such a shame as I had so much to do. The light's so bright now it hurts my eyes. It's peaceful.*

We had come to the end of the session so I brought Alex out of trance and she opened her eyes. She could understand the connection between her phobia and the horror of so much blood and death and also the horrific nature of her deaths in the lives she had just witnessed. She expressed relief that the regressions had finished as they had been intense but she also felt much calmer too.

Alex returned a week later to say that although she was still scared of needles and injections, she felt that there had been a reduction in the intensity of the fear; it didn't feel that it had as much energy in it as before our first regression session. She went into trance and was soon in her next past life, and as soon as she moved into it, she became anxious as she spoke to me:

> *I'm in an old-fashioned cobbled street and it's very busy and the sounds of lots of voices and carriages. There are women walking past wearing long dresses and bonnets. I'm a young boy, a street urchin, about 7 years old. I'm dirty and I don't have any shoes. I'm alone; this is a normal day for me. I steal something from a shop and as the shopkeeper shouts at me I run out of the shop into the street. I'm run over by a carriage; it all happens so quickly. I go under the wheel. I'm semi-conscious and I can hear voices as people start to gather round me. I've cracked my head at the back. I'm starting to feel sick — I can see blood and the torn tissues of my leg. I see the bone sticking up; it's come away from the knee. I can't feel anything in my right leg but there's pain in my right hip. I feel dizzy now.*

Alex paused as she grimaced at the scene she was reliving. Her breathing continued to come quickly and her eyes narrowed as she moved to the next part of the life. She gasped out the words:

> *They're cutting off my leg below the knee; I can't stop them. Someone's holding my shoulders. I can see the saw — it glistens.*

She continued to moan and writhe in the chair for a minute before she suddenly flopped down and sighed. Her face lost its tightness and her eyes relaxed:

> *I see white light now and I feel so much better. The light's bright. I feel safe, warm and looked after; I'm going up and up. I turn round and look down to see my body — a little boy; pale, skinny and dirty. I'm glad I'm going to the light; I feel that I'm being hugged. I can sense people around me but I can't see them.*

The life was over and although the end of the boy's life was a sad one, the chances are that it was a relief for him to have left such a tough existence. I have had quite a few clients who have been run over by horse-driven carriages and wagons in regression sessions; it seems to have been a regular form of death and injury in past times (especially in busy cities in the 1800s and early 1900s).

Alex's experience of going into the light after death is also a common one, with many people reporting similar things in thousands of sessions. As I mentioned in an earlier chapter, it appears that when we die, we leave our physical body and travel in our light body (or astral body) away from earth into the spirit world. This is a place in which we are able to heal and come to terms with the life we have just lived and prepare for our next incarnation. Some people just report receiving feelings of love once they have passed over, others describe spirit guides taking them to halls of learning in which they review the life they have just lived and learn were they went wrong.

Alex then moved into her fourth past life and this one contained more narrative than the others. She was an 18-year-old woman in Victorian or Edwardian times:

I'm walking alone in the countryside carrying a basket; it's a nice day. Someone is sick, one of the poor people. I think my father's the local doctor. I feel a real sense of injustice when I see the poverty and I'm angry that it's such a man's world. Father says I'm too headstrong. I can't let these people down through lack of food. I'm carrying some old-fashioned potions that I've made into a tea and some bread. I have some honey from our beehive. There are a lot of dirty children and one of them has a terrible cough. They can't afford to see a doctor. I feel an intense anger that people take no notice of the poverty. I go home and my father is stood there; we argue. He says that no daughter of his is going out and mixing with those people;

we're the talk of the village. I tell him that he should do more to help. He doesn't like that; I'm not supposed to talk back to him. He slaps me across my face and I just look at him in disgust. He says that it's about time I was married and off his hands. I don't think I have a mother; I didn't know her. He despatches me to my aunt in Coventry; he's sent me here to learn how to be a proper lady. At first it's fun; I'm in a ballroom and a young man holds my hand. I look up into his face with bright eyes. Later on I get pregnant. I'm laid in bed after childbirth; I can't move and I'm very tired and extremely pale. I keep falling asleep. They used clamps to pull the baby out and there was blood everywhere. I was screaming and then nothing. It's an effort to move. I can hear the baby crying but it seems a long way off. I haven't even seen it. A man's holding my hand. I keep drifting off. I feel sad but then I'm looking down from above and I can't feel any pain and I have no cares. I'm being pulled upwards and away. It's over.

With these words Alex breathed deeply and relaxed. We finished the session and once more she understood why she associated blood with pain and fear in her present life. Quite simply, her subconscious was saying to itself 'blood = death', so anytime in her present life she saw blood it triggered fears of death and the pain of dying.

When she arrived for her final session a few weeks later Alex told me that she was no longer getting any feelings of fear in her stomach when she was at work injecting people. She knew that the phobia was significantly reduced and she also felt calmer at work generally. Once she was in hypnosis her subconscious indicated that there were no more past lives that we had to explore, and it took her into a very upsetting memory in her present life that also had a direct connection to causing the phobia. She remembered being a young, newly qualified nurse working in a children's ward which had a very strict ward sister in charge. She was forced by the ward sister to give her first injection to an unwilling and scared child who was pinned down by the sister whilst she did it. She felt very apprehensive as she did this and 'the child screamed the place down' and could hardly walk afterwards. The needle had hit a nerve and she felt so guilty because she thought the child could have been paralysed. She couldn't relax for days afterwards and she couldn't sleep as she felt so traumatised.

We neutralised the fear that had been stored in this memory and Alex's subconscious took her into the final section of our work together, which she found even more surprising than the past life memories. She went back into the life of one of her great-great-grandmothers. In this case she mainly experienced the events in a disassociated state, watching in the third person the events happening to her ancestor (and I should mention that she knew nothing about her ancestor prior to the session):

> *She has auburn hair and green eyes; she has a sparkle in her eyes. She's in her kitchen reading the tea leaves for a soldier who's there. She's a strong person, very determined. I think she lives on Hessle Road.* (This, I should clarify, was the centre of Hull's fishing industry for generations. Many trawler men and their families lived there in a close-knit community. The men there were poor, tough and hard-drinking, and so too were many of the women. The streets were made up of back-to-back terraced houses and primitive living conditions. Hessle Road is a local byword for hardiness and stoicism under difficult living conditions.)
>
> *She's very caring, helps to deliver babies in other people's houses. Everybody knows everybody in the street. It's a hard life though, her hands are red with all the hard work, all the washing and scrubbing for five children. Something's happened at the docks. She's there with a man who's got a long piece of*

steel like a knife or a harpoon right through his eye. He's still alive but his eyeball is hanging out and he's covered in blood. She's coping with the sight but she feels useless, she doesn't know what to do. I can feel his grip getting tighter, as if he's holding my hand. It was a long piece of steel that was in his eye and it had gone through into the brain. He says to her "tell my missus" and soon after he dies. She's tough and tries to be in control but it bothers her and keeps coming back to her in her dreams. She's sat up in bed feeling angry with herself for being so stupid. It's as if she has to get on with life but it's still there, you just don't talk about it. She has a certain standing in the street and she can't appear to be weak. I can feel the fear in her stomach.

Alex was silent for some time and I could see that she was working through something by the look of concentration on her face so I didn't interrupt her inner process. Eventually she became a little bit emotional as she told me that something special was happening:

I have a feeling of being pushed back into my present life, but it's as if she's in my body. I feel her strength inside me, though I can also feel her fear and sadness. I'm hugging her and telling her that it's OK, I'm with her so she's not alone. It's OK for her to cry. I feel her tears but they've gone now and I'm left with her feelings of confidence and courage inside me. She's peaceful now, as if she's let go of something that had always troubled her.

Alex came out of trance feeling strong and powerful, as though she had brought back with her the ancestor's resources of fortitude and tenacity. It appeared that she had also healed her great-great-grandmother's trauma. Of course, she had died long before Alex was born but there is a Shamanic concept that our ancestors live on energetically long after they die physically, and it may be that our session had allowed the spirit of her great-great-grandmother to be laid to rest in some way. Of course I don't know for certain if this Shamanic concept is a reality or just a bit of wishful thinking, but I do know that Alex was no longer scared of needles and that she also felt much more confident as a result of our sessions together.

***

Eli was a 20-year-old store worker who initially came to me because she had a phobia of flying (aerophobia). However, once she sat in front of me in my office and started to talk about herself, she was much more troubled than I had expected. Not only did she have a fear of flying but she also had a constant state of anxiety as well as emetophobia (fear of vomit) and negative thoughts. As she was flying to America just a few weeks after our first session, I knew I only had a limited time that I could work with her, and although I guessed that all of her issues were interconnected, the flying phobia was the primary focus of our work together. As it happened though, as we worked on the flying phobia, we also did therapy on all of her issues in the three sessions in which I saw her.

Once I'd taken a history of her problems and her background, I took her into trance and asked her subconscious to indicate whereabouts the traumas were in the past that had caused the phobia, and it indicated that there was a past life and an ancestor's life that needed to be explored, as well as some events in this lifetime. I guided her back into the past life, which proved to be a highly unusual one. I asked her to tell me what she was experiencing in the past life, and she started to speak quietly:

I'm in the living room of an old house, it's the afternoon and I feel excited. I'm a woman, around 30 years old, and I'm cleaning and listening to music and waiting for someone who's coming home. It's someone I've not seen for a while. I get a sense of an airplane flying over the sea; it's a long trip in a big old plane. I'm waiting for my husband to come home; he's a passenger on the plane. It's as though I can see him looking out of a window on the plane. It's been a long flight and the weather is very bad so they have to make an emergency landing.

As Eli relived all of this she was very tense. What was strange was that she appeared to be experiencing the man's feelings, even though she was a woman in that life. As she continued sharing the life with me, she still seemed to be able to feel the man's feelings:

They land, far away in a foreign country in bad weather. It takes him days to come home using lots of small planes; some of the flights are even bumpier. He comes home though and he's OK. I feel such a relief now. I've been such a mess; when he didn't come home, I expected the worst. He's not scared of anything but he cries because he's so relieved to be home.

As she said this Eli became a little emotional. Something in the way that she was experiencing this past life felt curious to me, so I asked her subconscious if in that past life her and her husband were Twin Souls. Her subconscious indicated with a 'yes'. What this means is that in that lifetime one soul had split into two people alive on earth at the same time. The concept of Twin Souls is quite rare (sometimes it's known as 'Twin Flames') but I have had this happen a few times over the years in other regression sessions.

What this meant of course, is that to release the trauma from that past life she also had to re-experience it as the man! I guided her into *his* body and she started to relive his trauma. As she did so she was very tense:

> *I'm coming home from military service in a foreign country. I think I'm English. The flight is nice to start with and I fall asleep, but I'm awakened by bad turbulence — it's a bumpy ride. When the pilot announces that we'll have to make an emergency landing I feel very scared and I start to cry a little. There's luggage falling out everywhere and people are screaming. It's a rough landing. I just want to get home, and I have to use some small planes which are even bumpier; one of the planes is so small it only has two seats in each row. When I get home, I cry because I was so afraid that I'd lose my wife.*

Once more Eli became emotional, and after crying for a short time she sighed and relaxed in the chair. She told me that she just felt relieved now and calm. Those past lives were cleared of their negative energy and she came out of trance surprised by what she had experienced but feeling calmer.

In her next session Eli regressed into a lot of memories from this lifetime, all of which involved being sick and vomiting in some way, either memories when she herself was vomiting or when others were sick around her. As she relived these memories she was both very tense and upset, but she released the emotions and felt calmer about them. This, of course, is one of the major processes in regression therapy — that of going through the significant emotional events that had caused the emetophobia in order to empty the memories of their negative emotional charge. Once the memories are 'cleared' of the emotions, they no longer cause any problems to the client and the negative effects that they have had upon the client are neutralised.

The emetophobia was a core issue, and connected to the flying phobia because Eli was terrified that if she was on board an aeroplane and she started to vomit during the flight she was trapped; she had nowhere to run to in order to escape. The fear of being trapped is often a significant aspect of a flying phobia, as is a fear of dying. This last aspect came through in our session as I guided Eli into the life of an ancestor, from whom she had inherited trauma.

This ancestor turned out to be her father, and she relived her father's emotional pain at the death of *his* father. As she experienced this (as though she was in the body of her father, looking out at the world through *his* eyes) she relived being in the hospital after *his* father had had a stroke, nursing him as he lay paralysed for a few days before dying. She cried as she did so, crying the tears that her own father had bottled up and never released. She became even more emotional as she went even further back into her father's life, into his early childhood, as she relived the death of his mother when he was around 2 years old. As she lay crying, she realised that the death of his father had triggered the locked-in sadness from his mother's death that he had never allowed himself to feel.

Having let go of her father's locked-in grief, Eli became calm and I gave her some hypnotic suggestions that she could now be free of all those memories and the negative effects that they had had upon her, negative effects which were causing the phobia of flying. She came out of trance feeling very calm and much more relaxed when she thought about flying.

Our final session, a few days before her flight, was very successful too. In this session I used Advanced EFT on her, a free-flowing version of Emotional Freedom Technique that involved tapping on points on the body whilst she tuned into various aspects of flying and the phobia. As well as tapping whilst she tuned into the thought of flying, I specifically tapped on the three main aspects of a flying phobia: fear of being trapped (claustrophobia); fear of not being in control (she was a self-confessed 'control freak') and fear of dying. In Eli's case she also had a fear of her loved ones (i.e. her family) dying which we tapped on too. She began the session with the fear of flying around seven out of ten in terms of its intensity. As we tapped, she constantly yawned and sighed, a sure sign that the tapping was working as this signifies that she was letting go of tension, anxiety and fear. By the end of the session her fear level was zero out of ten. The phobia was cured. I taught her how to use EFT for herself so that she could keep working to tap down any residual feelings that might pop up before or during the flight, and she left my office feeling more relaxed than she had felt in a long time.

A few weeks later I received a text from Eli, confirming the success of the sessions:

'Made it to San Francisco on Tuesday! The flight went surprisingly well; think the appointments we had worked.'

Upon her return I also received the following text:

'Got back on Sunday, everything went well. I think our appointments were a good idea and worked very well!'

I think I can add these texts to the drawer-full of postcards I've received over the years from clients with flying phobias who got to their holiday destinations without any problems and who were overjoyed that their flights were stress-free!

Chapter 19

'Foul Is Fair, and Fair Is Foul' (or the Terrible Fate of Witches)

Over the years, in the thousands of past life regression sessions I have overseen I have found that there are 'themes' which crop up time after time. The most obvious is that it is so often the death in a previous life which is causing the client's problem in this life (I estimate that at least 60% of Past Life Therapy concerns releasing death traumas); another is that of rape which features regularly in former lives. I have also facilitated hundreds of sessions in which clients have been persecuted as witches. It appears that in Western Europe and America, for a couple of centuries at least, there was a religion-fuelled madness during which tens of thousands of people (mainly women and girls) were tortured and brutally killed for allegedly being witches. The insane drive to brutalise females in this way was instigated, not surprisingly, by the Christian Church, and any woman could be put on trial and murdered simply by being accused of being a witch. Here are a handful of such cases…

Liv, a Norwegian woman in her 60s, came to me suffering from extreme anxiety. She described it as being a constant heavy feeling which had been in her chest, neck and shoulders all day, every day, for several years. I asked her to describe the feelings and without realising she used words that immediately suggested to me that there was a past life involved somewhere. 'It feels as if something is tying me up across my chest', she said, words which, as you will see, connected to the first past life that we entered.

I have sometimes found that when a client describes their issue, especially if it is a physical problem or one that manifests itself in their body, that they unwittingly describe something that directly connects to the trauma in a past life that has caused their problem. One man with constant headaches said that he felt 'like I've been shot in the head with a musket ball'. And guess what, in a previous life he had died in the English Civil Wars by being shot in the head (with, of course, a musket ball). A lady with back pain described it as 'like someone sticking a knife in my back'. Someone else said that their Irritable Bowel Syndrome stomach pain felt 'like I've been speared'. And guess what? Yes, you've got it, they'd both died in this way in past lifetimes.

So when Liv said that it felt like she'd been tied up, I guessed there'd be something similar in a past life. I didn't say anything though, as I didn't want to lead her in any way. I actually expected that some of her anxiety would be caused by the number of deaths to close family members that she had experienced in this current lifetime, but I was surprised when her subconscious signalled (once she had entered trance, using the IMR signal) that there were no traumas in this life but there were several past lives and some ancestral trauma causing the anxieties.

She moved firstly into the life of one of her great-great-grandfathers, four generations ago. Throughout the regression, she was a little emotional and breathing in a distressed way as she shared with me the traumas as if she was in the body of her great-great-grandfather:

> *I'm in a fishing boat on the sea in the middle of a big storm. The sky's black and there are big waves. I'm in charge of the boat. The storm came out of nothing. I'm so scared; we can't make this. I feel heaviness in my chest; there are some of the men in the water. I can't help them; I feel so sad for those young boys, they have wives and children at home. Many of them are in the water, shouting. I can't breathe and my shoulders feel as if they are hunched up. I feel the shame and I'm so sad that I can't help*

> *them. I'm in the water now, besides the boat, my hands feel so numb. I feel sadness and shame in my hands, shoulders and heart. I see the light now; I'm starting to feel calm.*

Liv breathed deeply and relaxed. Her ancestor had obviously died and she had released the fear and guilt that had been passed down to her from him, feelings that were locked in her body causing her anxieties. Although this was a standard regression session, in which we released negative emotions to clear a problem in this lifetime, there is an unusual feature here which may need to be explained.

You may ask, how can an ancestor pass down *death* trauma to another generation? It makes sense to acknowledge that traumas can be passed down through the genes. For example, if a trauma happens in your mother's life before you were born then that trauma can be transmitted genetically into you. But how could the death of her great-great-grandfather come down in that way, as he was dying and couldn't physically pass it down through the family genes?

When I first began working with ancestral trauma in regression, I believed that the only way in which the trauma was passed down was via the genes, but occasionally a client would explore a trauma (in the same way as Liv) which couldn't possibly be handed down in that way. It appears that it doesn't have to be transmitted physically, but it is a form of energy that is passed down in some way outside of the physical. How this happens I don't know and I can't explain it scientifically, but I have a feeling that it connects in some way to the strange world of quantum physics.

I allowed Liv to relax for a couple of minutes before I asked her to move to something else that was causing her anxiety state, and soon she was in a past life:

> *I'm alone in an old timber hut. I'm a woman, around* 23 *years old, and I'm wearing a long white dress. I feel tense, as if I'm*

waiting for something to happen. I'm listening and I can hear a lot of people coming and they're shouting. They want me. I'm saying that I haven't done anything wrong, but they say that I'm a witch because of the medicines that I make. They're laughing as they destroy everything — all of the herbal medicines that I make. Many of these people I have helped in the past; I feel betrayed. They take me out of the hut and burn it and take me to a town where there are many people. How can they be like this when I have helped them? No-one will listen to me; they put me in a prison cell for several days. I know what's happened — I was helping a man who had a sick wife. She's very sick and I know that I can't help her. She's angry and accuses me of wanting to kill *her because I want her man. But I don't, I just can't help her.*

Liv started to cry and her voice sounded more and more desperate as she went on:

I feel a big pain in my heart. Her husband believes her and after she died he accuses me of killing her and he'll tell that to the authorities. I have pain all over my body. She was always jealous of me. It feels so bad to be accused of something I didn't do. I'm in the prison and I feel so sad. I know I'm going to die; I just give up. She started to shake and breathe rapidly; her body twisted as if she was trying to get away and she gasped out her words:

They take me to the water, put me in a boat and row me out onto the water. My hands and feet are tied. A rope is round my chest so I can't move my arms. There are many people watching. I ask them to defend me but they don't; I have helped so many of them. I'm so angry, how can they do this to me? In my head I'm promising myself that I'll never use this knowledge again. I'm staring at a man who's guarding me in the boat — I helped him too but he pushes me into the water; it's dark water and I have no chance. Liv continued to kick and writhe for a few seconds before she suddenly relaxed and she was calm:

I see the light and I feel calm as I float above everything. It's finished.

Although the life was over, I asked her if there was anything else that she needed to be aware of, and she told me that the woman who had been treated and said that she'd wanted to kill her was intensely angry, firing real hate at her in the past life. She cursed Liv and wanted the worst for her forever, which shocked Liv as she was only trying to help her. We did some work to release the curse and to send it back with love from whence it came, and once this was done and Liv felt that it had been laid to rest, she came out of trance.

I'm never sure about curses; in other words how real and effective they actually are. I have colleagues who place much store in the reality of curses and believe that a curse can affect someone over many lifetimes, but I don't know if this is really possible. However, just to be on the safe side I treat them seriously and if one comes through in a regression session, I usually work to neutralise it.

Once we had talked the session through in order to de-brief, Liv left my office and returned a few weeks later. She told me that since our session she had felt quite anxious a lot of the time, which meant that her subconscious was already bringing the next 'layer' of anxiety to the surface, ready for us to work on. In this case, the next layer of 'stuff' was two more previous lives. Both were quite unusual:

I'm a young woman in my 20s and I'm walking alone down a street with cobblestones and it's the evening. I feel that I'm poor. My father owns a pub; it's a smelly, dirty place and I'm going there to help serve beer. I don't like to be there. He hasn't much money and he has trouble paying for things. I get there but he isn't there and I don't know where he is. I feel afraid because he's always there. I have no mother so I'm on my own. He doesn't come back that night and so I run the pub. He doesn't return at all and I'm left to run the pub and it's a hard life. There are many poor people in the streets. Sometime later a man tells me that my father has been kidnapped and killed by body snatchers. They do this in the name of science. It's done by some men in the pub; they make money from it. It's so unfair as I have no money and I have to stay as I have nothing else. I feel hopeless and I never feel that I can trust anyone. I'm there for many years and finally I die in my 50s. I'm sick and alone and I know that I'm going to die; I'm ready to die and it's a relief when I go.

Real Burke and Hare stuff, eh? I've never had anything related to body snatching in all of my sessions so that's why I said that this was quite unusual. What was normal though was the poverty and hopelessness felt by Liv, something that occurs regularly in past life sessions.

Liv relaxed for a while and then told me that she was standing alone in the dark in a forest:

> *I'm a man in my late 20s. I can hear wolves howling. I know the wolves; I'm listening to who it is that's howling. I'm not afraid as they are my friends. I listen so I can find where they are. I find them; they're a family and they're so happy to see me. I make a fire and sleep there. I feel safe; it's so calm and beautiful to be with them.* Liv had a smile on her face and she was calm and happy. I asked her to move to the next significant part of that life and after a few seconds she became deeply emotional. Between her sobs she choked out:
>
> *I came back another time to find them all dead. They were my best friends and they've been shot and killed for their skins. It's a terrible sight to see their bodies after they've been*

skinned. I dig their grave and just sit crying, it's so unfair. I feel guilty because I told someone that I had these wolves as friends and they followed me to find where they were. If it wasn't for me, they would have lived. I feel grief everywhere in my body. One of them I called Shakira and I can't bear that she's gone. I sit and mourn and then build a small hut nearby from timber; I want to be there. I live alone and become a friend to many animals but I never forget the wolves. I live in nature for many years and die there as an old man. I die sitting on their graves, it's OK to go. I feel relief as I see the bright light. I can see Shakira waiting for me.

Liv's tears turned to calmness and the smile on her face told me that she had let go of the guilt of that lifetime. She came back to full awareness and told me that the anxiety that had been inside her for years had evaporated away. She felt at peace. The negative emotions of anxiety, fear and guilt that had caused her to come to me for help had been discharged and she was able to get on with her life as if they had never been there.

***

Tracy came to me with severe anxieties. She'd been getting panic attacks for many years but for the previous four years they had become stronger and more frequent. We found that there were two past lives causing them. In the first, she was a street urchin, a young girl living rough on the streets and scavenging to stay alive after her parents died and left her homeless. In the second, she was a young woman running barefoot through trees on the edge of a lake:

I'm running away from people; I don't feel scared as I'm confident that I can get away. I hide in the trees and bushes and listen. The people from the village are all after me but they'll have a job catching me though. They think I'm a witch; I'm not, I just have feelings about things that are going to happen. I hear voices so I run through the trees; I know I can get away. They're getting closer but I know I've got somewhere to hide. I've got away again. I knew I would. I'm hiding in a trench covered with trees. How much longer can I keep on running? They caught up with me once and threw me in the lake and threw stones at me. That was a warning. They've gone now. I can't go back to the village in daylight so I go to stay with an old couple who are friends. I'm always going to be an outcast. I'm not ready to be caught yet.

As she narrated this Tracy was relatively calm, but she then became tense and she started to cry. She was choking as if she couldn't get her breath and shifting around in the chair:

They've caught me. I thought I could get away. They tie me up and they're laughing and cheering as they throw me into the lake. As I'm drowning, they throw things at me. I'm at peace now, it's over.

Tracy came out of trance feeling relief and peaceful. The anxieties had gone and when I saw her again five months later, she told me that she hadn't had a single panic attack. What's more, she said that her insecurities about going to new and unknown places had gone too – she had even been on the London Eye and enjoyed it!

***

Pam was in her early 40s but she was struggling with severe psoriasis which covered many parts of her body. I have found that all skin problems are caused by locked-in anger. This means that the person is holding onto a high degree of anger which is coming out through the skin. Anger is a composite emotion, which means that it always has another emotion underneath it. Sometimes this underlying emotion is fear, but more often than not it is sadness (I usually know that a client is starting to clear their locked-in anger when they begin to cry). Once she was in trance her subconscious indicated that the cause of her anger was one past life, and within seconds she went into the life and started talking to me:

> *I'm a woman, around 50, and I'm alone in a forest. I live in a small hut there and I'm cooking in a pot over a fire. I feel lonely because everyone is frightened of me; they think that I'm a witch. I'm not a witch, I just like living in nature. I love being surrounded by trees, plants and animals, they're my friends. I have no human friends and people don't want to be around me and rumours are spreading about me. Children throw stones at my hut. I feel helpless so I lock myself away. Everyone's against me and I'm scared they'll do something to hurt me as they hate me so much.*

So far Pam had spoken with a depth of misery in her voice, but then she jerked as if shocked and she began to cry:

> *They've come for me; they're going to kill me. They're outside my house; I can't get away, there are so many of them. I don't want to die. There's no point in running or fighting, they've already made their minds up. There's no-one to help me. They've tied my hands together. I've done nothing wrong, I've done nothing wrong.'* With desperation in her voice she started to shout: *'I'VE DONE NOTHING WRONG. I'M NOT A WITCH'*. Tears were flowing down her cheeks and her voice was panic-stricken; she looked terrified:
>
> *They put me on a cart pulled by two horses; they're all excited that they've got the witch and they take me into the town and parade me through the streets. It's a horrible place*

and it stinks. I live in a beautiful place; I just want to be there. My red hair makes me different too. They're shouting and throwing things at me — "witch, witch". I'm not a witch. They take me to the side of a river and drag me to a wooden chair-type thing. They strap me in. I feel scared. A man wearing a big black hat with a buckle on it with hair curled under it like a woman's is shouting questions at me. He's dressed in black and white clothes and he's saying "you are the Devil; you are a witch". He's asking me over and over again if I'm a witch and I'm saying that I'm not a witch. He says that if I admit it my soul will go to Heaven, otherwise I'll be with the Devil forever. People are laughing and cheering, it's like a celebration. The chair goes into the water and they hold me under the water. I feel like my lungs will burst. They keep pushing me under and the more I say "no" the longer I'm under the water. He says that if I admit it they'll stop but I'm not with the Devil.

At this stage Pam was sobbing and twisting around in the chair, her head tilted upwards as if she was trying to breathe, her hands were gripping the arms of the chair and her feet kicking as she gasped out the words:

I want it to stop and I'm getting weak, I can't fight anymore. He's asked me again, I can't breathe, I've no strength left, I'm going to die. I say "yes" as I don't want it to go on any longer. I go under and I feel my lungs filling with water. I stop struggling. I feel peaceful and free.

Her body went limp and she started to relax and breathe normally. The life was almost over and quietly she gave a poignant tailpiece to the experience:

I'm floating above and I can see they drag my body out of the water and cut off my hair and then they throw it on a fire.

> *They're all cheering and dancing around. I can see my mother's come, she's been waiting for me; they burnt her too and killed her.*

Although Pam came out of hypnosis feeling exhausted, she also felt very peaceful. She now understood why her body had created the skin problem; although she did get even more understanding about her life. This was why, she explained, she had always felt like an outsider. In her teens at school she had often felt terrified; panicking so much at times that she was even unable to learn. She had felt unimportant and scared that the other kids would laugh at her if she spoke. So many things about her life began to make sense, she said. These insights, together with the release of the energies from the past life, meant that she could finally begin to heal physically and emotionally.

***

In her 40s, when I treated her for her alcoholism, Linda had also been blind for a number of years after contracting meningitis. She had been drinking a litre of spirits every day for months to alleviate stress and as well as being blind she had a number of health problems. In our first session we discussed her emotional state and the traumas in her life. I took her into trance and got an IMR (which told me that there were some past lives as well as ancestor's lives that needed working through) and gave her some post-hypnotic suggestions to start taking control of her drink problem.

This she duly did, as when she returned a week later, she hadn't had any alcohol since I saw her. She was feeling calmer and (as I had asked her to do) she was drinking more water so she felt better physically. Obviously, this was a good start but I knew that if we didn't work on the underlying emotional causes to her unhappiness and stress she would probably go back to drinking at some stage in the future. Her first past life was the one in which she was alleged to be a witch:

> *I'm a woman, around 40 years old and I'm helping a woman to give birth. I save the lives of the mother and the baby but people don't understand that I'm only trying to help. They don't like me and what I do scares them. This sort of thing has happened before when doctors can't save them and I have. Women come to see me in secret to help them to conceive. I work with herbs and I see things that others don't see — in my head I saw the boy fall into the lake and die a few weeks before it actually happened. I feel like a freak; I wish I wasn't like this; I just want to be the same as everybody else. They point fingers at me and say I'm a witch. I'm only trying to help people. I remember when I was a 7-year-old girl. My mother loves me very much and is protective of me. We don't have much but I'm happy as she loves me. Other people don't like us but I don't understand as I'm only little. They shout at mum in the streets but she says not to listen. Mum makes things out of plants, there are all sorts growing in the kitchen. People come and go regularly, often they cry but mum makes them better. One day they knock on the door and I watch them take her out and tie her to a post and they stone her; she dies. I feel so sad. My father won't allow me to talk about it. I'm not allowed to talk about the things that I see either; he says it's very naughty and I've got to start thinking about what's real and what isn't real. He cuts all my hair off as a punishment because I'm like my mother. I'm scared and I want my mum. I still talk to her even though she's not around but I'm not allowed to do that; if he catches me I get put outside in the yard and it's very cold. As I grow up, I learn to keep my thoughts to myself but nobody knows that I still talk to my mum. Dad doesn't beat me as much and he drinks a lot. I give him mugs of beer and it stops him treating me badly. He falls asleep and I sit in front of the fire and talk to my friends*

in the spirit world. When I'm 16 it all comes out into the open. I see that my best friend will go out with friends in the future and that she doesn't come back. I tell her and she's scared so she tells her parents. Everyone's talking, saying that I'm just like my mother. A few months later my friend goes out and she's murdered and everyone's angry with me. I run away and I'm cold as I have nowhere to stay. I feel sad and scared, I'm an outcast and everyone thinks I'm strange. I have to grow up and rebuild my life. I keep plodding through life until someone finds out and I have to move on. I spend most of my life moving on. I take my mother's herbs with me and help people who are in need but they soon turn on me. Making people better makes me feel good.

Linda was silent as she moved through time. I guessed that the inevitable was going to happen, and sure enough she began to cry and shake as she spoke:

Some of them are outside my home calling me names and telling me to leave town. I'm sad and scared. Some of these people have been to me for help in the past. They're plotting against me. I wake that night to find my thatched roof is on fire. I run outside and they're waiting. They tie me up and take me into the village. I'm so cold. They leave me tied up outside for days and they're all laughing at me. I just want to die, I'm so cold. Some of them throw things at me. I helped them so much. I'm giving up, I'm weak and cold and shivering. I just wish they'd finish it so I can be warm. After a few days they come for me at night but I can't walk. They take me to the water; a lot of people are shouting and laughing. They stand me up and then throw me in. I can't breathe.

At this point Linda was coughing and choking as she experienced drowning, and then she softened and lay quietly. She told me that she was calm and floating upwards and leaving the life behind. I gave her some suggestions for feeling relaxed and that the negative effects that the past life had had upon her would now be dissolved away, leaving her feeling free. She came out of trance and despite the horrors that she had experienced she smiled as she knew that she had let go of something that had always held her back and caused problems throughout her life.

Although these three examples of clients being killed as witches all ended with them being drowned, I have had many other clients who were accused of witchcraft in past lives who were horribly tortured, hung, stoned, burnt to death or strangled. The consequences of these horrific deaths are many and varied, from anxiety and phobias to depression, lack of confidence, trust issues and even physical problems in this present life.

One lady who was very psychic and who wanted to become a professional clairvoyant was terrified of sitting in front of a person to give them a reading. This caused her much conflict as a part of her was eager to do so, but the thought of someone looking at her whilst she told them their future caused her to shake and panic. We found that she had died horribly in two past lives as a witch, in one of them she had had her tongue cut out before being brutally killed.

I often find that clients who have psychic abilities, are the ones who have had past lives where they were accused of witchcraft and persecuted. In almost all of these cases they were not witches at all but herbal healers or they had the gift of seeing the future.

***

These are just a few cases from my files in which clients have found that they have experienced past lives in which they were accused of being witches and brutally punished. I'd like to end this chapter by moving away from the 'witchy' theme and share with you more of Linda's experiences in regression, as her other previous lives were unusual too. In one of them she was a tribal Medicine Man or Witch Doctor, feeling the heavy burden of responsibility that came with his position in the tribe. I think her third former life that we explored is even more interesting. In this, she saw herself as a nun working in Victorian times in a children's hospital:

> *I feel calm and peaceful and although I'm tired I have all the patience in the world for these lovely children; they all love me. I'm in the right place in my life and I feel a lot of joy. It's a simple life and I adore the children. The hospital is near the convent. My only regret is that I never had children of my own, but in one way I have one big family. Some of the children I looked after in my early years are now having their own children. I've been a nun for over twenty years since I was 14. I spend a lot of time in the hospital garden praying for the children; I don't care for the convent and its stuffy ways. I know my mission in life is to help heal the children. I don't always follow the rules and regulations; I do what's right when I feel it's right. I don't understand why we should sit in a cold chapel when we can be outside seeing the beauty of life.*

Linda had a beatific smile on her face throughout all of this; I asked her to move to the next significant part of the life and straight away she looked serious and troubled:

> *I'm on the ward and a lady who's very ill is giving birth. I'm attending her and the baby. She's having a terrible time and the baby's very sick. I can't do much; I just wrap the baby up. The pain and terror in the mother's face is awful to see. The weather's terrible outside. I'm waiting for the priest to come to give the last rites to the baby. The parents ask me to pray for the baby. I lay my hands on its tiny body and pray for it*

to be at peace and out of pain. As I hold the baby suddenly it's peaceful and it's not fighting anymore; it's breathing better and looking better. I pass him to the mother and the doctor says to me "you're a miracle worker". Later, when everything has settled, I go for a long walk; I'm overflowing with love. The next day everybody knows about the miracle worker; I didn't know that it would be one of the saddest days of my life. Parents surround me, wanting me to pray for their children. Then I make my second mistake. I prayed for a very sick girl and she got better. Word goes round. I pray for an old nun, a very spiritual lady, dying of old age. She says that I am a saint and I have to use the gift that I've been given. The priest and others hear her and want to know what I've been doing. After that I don't have a moment alone. I feel sad and exhausted and I miss my peaceful times in the garden. I don't want this anymore. People send me gifts of jewellery and money but I send them back. I just want my peace and my time with the children back. The priest says that I can't stay there any longer as the hospital is full of children and adults hoping for my healing. People are coming to the convent offering gold and silver, so he tries to make a deal with me; I can pray with visitors and they make donations to the convent. I decline as I don't want that, I just want to work on the children's ward. I decide that I want to be sent overseas. I pack my things and I feel so sad. I dearly miss the children and my garden. Now I just live in despair. Why has God forsaken me? I'm not sure anymore if there is a God. I'm on the ship, near the bottom of the ship, and it's very smelly. I get sick. I just lay there for days with a dry mouth and a high temperature. I'm so tired and hot and I can't stop shaking.

At this stage Linda was breathing with difficulty and moaning. She started to cry:

I miss my children so much, and the beauty of my life there. I feel so weak. There are rats running around too. They're eating my flesh. I can't get up, I need to get out but I can't get up.

Slowly Linda started to breathe normally and relaxed. With a new smile on her face she spoke softly:

I feel lovely, I'm floating. I'm warm and I'm in the light.

The life was over, and I felt the poignancy of the sad waste of a life that had so much to offer other people, especially children. As I write about this past life it strikes me that this is exactly the type of past life experience in regression that past life 'deniers' find difficult to explain away. I have often faced criticism from people who say that all previous lives that my clients experience are made up; that they are purely imaginary. They say that everyone in past lives claims to have lived in Egypt or to have been famous historical people. They say that everyone in past lives says that they are Native Americans or that their lives are dramatic or they are heroes in battle. I hope that what you've read already in this book will allow you to see that these accusations are actually not the case. Yes, some people experience previous lives as Egyptians and Native Americans, but very, very few appear to have been famous in any way. And most past life regressions are actually quite uneventful, with very little in the way of dramatic events at all.

Linda's former life as the nun is hardly the sort of thing that anyone is going to make up. Surely, if she was going to imagine a past life, she would have imagined something more theatrical. And also, why would she want to imagine such a past life in order to help her with her drinking problem? The obvious thing to have made up would be to create a past life as a drunkard, maybe someone who dies as a result of alcoholism, not the story of a nun whose life goes wrong as a result of her healing powers.

Looking at this from another angle, I have also heard it said by another past life therapist that one thing that goes towards *proving* the reality of the past life experience is the tiny, maybe insignificant details that a client reports when they're in trance. Here in Linda's story was one such aside: 'The weather's terrible outside'. Small details such as that are not usually reported by someone who is just making up an imaginary life in their head. I should also say that having facilitated thousands of past life regressions, that if someone is just imagining a past life that the quality of it is so different to a 'real' past life. There is a fantasy element to it that stands out to a trained observer. And by the way, I've yet to meet anyone who criticises the concept of past life regression who has observed, attended or experienced a substantial number of past life sessions. Most of them just make a bigoted judgement based on prejudice, not on evidence or experience.

Also, few of my clients come to me with a belief in, or knowledge of, reincarnation. They are often very surprised when their subconscious (using the IMR) signals that there are past life causes to their issues and takes them into a past life. As well as this I regularly see clients who deny the reality of past lives, often having a strong disbelief in the afterlife. Why does their IMR finger so often rise when I ask if there any past life causes? I had a top London barrister, a practising Roman Catholic brought up in a strictly Catholic household, come to me with a severe alcohol problem. He was a functioning alcoholic, able to work every day in a highly stressful environment, but who every night of the week was drinking until he was completely smashed. He had been forced to come to see me by his partner whose alcoholism had been cured when we worked in her past lives. He sat in front of me in my office and told me, somewhat aggressively as he was used to getting his own way, that all that past life stuff I'd done with his partner was total bunkum and there was no way on this earth was I to try any of that malarkey with him. Imagine his surprise when he was in trance and I asked his IMR if there were any past lives connected to causing the emotional pain that was being anaesthetised by the alcohol, and the IMR finger shot up in the air to say 'Yes'! He was even more surprised when his subconscious took him into a past life in the French Revolution and he experienced the life of a French aristocrat who lost the love of his life! Again, if past lives were not real this would surely never have happened?

I've also heard it said that there are no such things as past life experiences, that they are actually the lives of our ancestors that are being relived in trance. As you have seen, I readily acknowledge that we can regress into the lives of ancestors in our bloodline, but I disagree that all past lives are simply ancestor's lives. If this was the case, why does the clients' subconscious differentiate between past lives and ancestor's lives? When my client is in trance and their subconscious is signalling using an Ideo-Motor Response, I ask if there are any traumas causing their problem in this life, past lives *and* ancestor's lives? For example, the subconscious will specifically indicate two past lives *and* an ancestor's life. Surely it wouldn't do this if past lives were not real; it would not signal when I asked 'past lives' and it would only signal when I asked 'ancestor's lives'.

As well as this, in almost all cases if a client experiences a 'recent' past life (i.e. the life before their present incarnation) that past life will not be in their current life family line.

All I can say is that I'm convinced that if a sceptic were to sit in my therapy sessions day after day, week after week, month after month and see my client's experiences, and the amazing healings and transformations that take place because of re-experiencing their past lives, they would soon change their tune and have a more open mind about the whole phenomenon.

Anyway, back to Linda. As a result of our sessions so far, she found that she had much more control over her drinking; she had hardly touched a drop of alcohol for weeks and rarely felt the desire for it. As well as this she felt calmer and more confident too. Our final regression that was connected to the alcohol problem, and which completely released her from her need for alcohol, was back into the life of one of her ancestors. This proved to be very traumatic and deeply unpleasant; once she was in hypnosis, she entered the life of one of her maternal great-grandmothers three generations ago:

> *I'm a young woman standing alone inside a chapel. My clothes are scratchy and uncomfortable. I feel cold but also tormented. My husband has become an alcoholic. There was an accident at a pond and our child drowned. My husband was there and he couldn't save him so he blames himself. He turned to alcohol because of the guilt and he hasn't left the house since that day, he just sits and drinks. I'm grieving the loss of two souls. I have strange feelings, half torment and half excitement as I'm waiting in the graveyard for someone. A man turns up and I'm really pleased to see him but I'm also tormented by my feelings for him. We're having an affair so I feel guilty but he makes me so happy; he's so kind. He's called Peter. He wants me to go away with him but I'm held back by my marriage vows and I'm torn between happiness and sadness.*

As Linda was silent for a short time her smiling face changed into one of tension and she started to shiver. With graveness in her voice she continued:

> *I'm back at my house now. I can't get in as the door's locked. It's cold and raining and I feel as if I've left my happiness behind me. It's very cold and I'm sitting in the outside toilet waiting for him to let me in. I want to go with Peter and leave this all behind but I'm scared of hell and damnation. My father's a man of the cloth and I'm scared of spending eternity in hell. Sometimes my husband gets so drunk he beats me up and then*

he forgets about it the next day. I just cover up the bruises. If God was a loving God, wouldn't he want me to be happy? Jesus was a kind man. Why is the Bible so contradictory? I know it's wrong what I'm doing but Peter loves me so much. He wants to take me to Ireland to start a new life together. Do I follow the Path of Righteousness or the Path of Happiness?

Suddenly Linda's body jerked and she put her hands up in front of her face, as if trying to protect herself. She was crying and her head jerked violently to one side, as if she'd been hit in the face:

He's come out of the house and he's beating me. Now he's locked me in the outside toilet for the night. He banged my head and I'm so cold. This is the final time; he's never going to do this to me again. I might just as well go to hell, at least it's warm there. I've made up my mind; I'm living in hell anyway so what's the difference? The next day I meet Peter at the chapel and he wants an answer; it's now or never. He's been patient with me. I walk away with him with just the clothes that I'm wearing. He takes me away; he's so in love with me and tender and kind and passionate. At first he's angry because of the bruises on my body, and even though I'm happy the fear of going to hell is never far away.

Linda started to calm down and was quiet for a while, indicating that she was moving through the life. Eventually she spoke and she sounded happy:

I'm in a garden in Ireland; it's a couple of years after I left my husband. I feel peaceful and I now have no regrets about leaving him. Now all the fear has gone from my life I feel closer to God the Creator of the Universe than ever before. Peter and I are very happy and excited that I'm pregnant. I feel a bit overwhelmed by the responsibility of looking after a child but I have a great love for it. I couldn't cope with the grief of losing another child. We're preparing together for the child; on an evening he's making a cot and I'm sewing. I'm excited and being careful with what I eat. It's a lovely day and I'm rubbing my tummy and singing to the baby as I feel it kicking. I can feel stomach pains; it's close to the birth time. I go for a short walk and suddenly I see my father; he's been searching for me and he's tracked me down. I don't know whether to rush to him or run away. I'm startled and I can feel my heart pumping. I feel scared as I can see that he's very angry. I'm hoping he'll forgive me now that I'm pregnant. I start to feel pain in my stomach. He's shouting at me, tells me that I'm going to hell for the shame I've brought on him. He's hitting me and crying as he screams at me. He pushes me over and I fall and bang my head on a metal railing. I can taste blood in my mouth and I feel dizzy and there's a pain in my head.

Once more she started to react and grimace and her hands were over her head as if she was trying to fend off blows. She was crying and groaning as she continued:

I'm on the ground and he's kicking me. I feel terrible pains in my stomach. He kicks me in the chest and stomach. He's sobbing and wailing, shouting that I'm shameful and a whore and I'm going to hell. My head hurts, my stomach hurts and I'm coughing up blood. I'm unconscious and later Peter finds me. The baby is born but I die; he calls her Lily after me. He's crying. I can't leave them, so I stay around in Spirit for a long time to look after her.

Linda was crying throughout all of this, but eventually she relaxed and then a quizzical look came upon her face. She began to talk once more as herself, not as her great-grandmother:

> *I was called Lily too; it's one of my names. My great-grandmother stayed around to look after me, and I think she's still around now. I was aware of her around me as I grew up. I can feel her in the room with us now. Maybe she can move on now.*

We realised that this ancestor had been unable to leave this earth plane because of the trauma of her death and also that she feared (because of her religious upbringing) that she would go to hell. I too could feel the presence of a spirit in the room (the air around where Linda lay in the chair was very cold). Together, Linda and I gently told her that it was now time for her to go home, that there was no such place as hell, that she was not going to be judged but she was going to a place of love and light, and that it was likely that Peter and Lily would be there waiting for her. As we did this, the atmosphere in the room changed and it became warm again and Linda said that she could feel that her great grandmother had finally been laid to rest. She came out of trance relieved and happy that she had let go of so much trauma. She didn't know anything about her family history as it was never spoken about by her parents, but she understood why she had felt so stressed during her life and why she had needed alcohol to soften the stress. She also knew that she was now free of the need to drink alcohol, something that remains with her to this day, ten years after our sessions together.

Chapter 20

'Alas!' said she, 'We Ne'er Can Be Made Happy by Compulsion!'

— Coleridge

One of the strangest, and sometimes difficult things for a therapist to work with, is that of Obsessive-Compulsive Disorder (OCD). This takes the form of someone having chronic and uncontrollable recurring thoughts (obsessions) or behaviours that they feel the need to repeat over and over again. These compulsions can take many forms and interfere with daily activities and usually cause significant distress. One of the most common forms of OCD is handwashing. Someone with OCD linked to handwashing (often connected to a fear of germs or of being contaminated in some way) will obsessively wash their hands many times each day, probably exaggerating the procedure of hand washing so that it lasts for several minutes. One of my OCD clients had such a terror of contamination that she would wash her hands at least 36 times a day, often for 10 or 15 minutes at a time. She had done this for such a long time that she had no top layer of skin on her hands, which were red raw; as a result she had to wear light gloves all the time. She would obsessively clean her house for hours (before she went out for the day, she would spend two or three hours cleaning) and if her husband so much as touched a door handle, she would immediately grab a handful of tissues and clean it. They were spending hundreds of pounds every month on tissues alone, which meant that her husband was unable to retire as they couldn't afford to do so. I dread to think how much she was spending on cleaning materials too.

Admittedly, that's one of the most extreme cases I have witnessed, but even milder OCD is a torment to the sufferer, not to mention embarrassing. One young girl came to me with a habit of needing to tap six times on the floor with her foot every time she was about to go through a doorway, and then six times again on the other side of the door once she'd gone through. She had done her best to hide it at work but someone in the office noticed her doing it one day and after that word went round about her affliction. Everyone in the office would stop work as soon as they saw her approaching a door and watched in fascination as she went through her little ritual. Shame is something that all OCD sufferers have to live with on a daily basis.

I mentioned trichotillomania earlier on in the book, a condition in which a person pulls their hair out all the time. I treated one woman with this who had no hair at all on the top of her head; she just kept a ring of hair around the sides, back and front so that when she wore a beret it looked like she had hair. She came for her first session and she looked quite normal, wearing a beret and short hair dangling down from it. When she took the beret off, I nearly screamed with the shock! The top of her head was completely bald. She looked like a medieval monk!

Another young woman with trichotillomania was obsessed about shaving her legs. She would spend hours in the bathroom if she was going for a night out with her boyfriend, and even after she had finished shaving her legs many times, she would still spend hours checking her legs with tweezers.

All of this would sound comical as it's so bizarre, but the tragedy is that for a person with OCD it makes their life a living hell.

Another common form of OCD is that of checking things over and over. We all check that we have turned the gas off or locked the door more than once, but my next client had the checking ritual to the 'nth' degree, as well as several other obsessions. John was a 20-year-old who was about to start working in a prison, and he knew that if he didn't get some help with his behaviours that he would not be able to keep the job. He first learnt some compulsions from his mum, who (when he was a young child) would shout at him to turn off the lights and electric sockets at home in case they started a fire. As a result around the age of 7 he too started switching everything off and then checking and re-checking many times that he had done so. Round the age of 11 he also started to check every night at bedtime that all the doors and windows at home were locked. Soon after he added in the ritual of holding up door handles so that they wouldn't droop down and checking and re-checking that the taps were turned off. He had many rituals before bed every night, and everything on the shelves in his bedroom had to be in exactly the same place – woe betide his mum if she cleaned his bedroom and moved anything even a millimetre out of line. He developed a fear of the number three or multiples of three; he then had to use the number eleven or multiples of eleven to neutralise the fear. He went through a phase of sniffing his fingers constantly in case they smelled of copper. He used to blink a lot, but this then turned into a nervous sniff and clearing his throat constantly.

The poor lad was obviously a bundle of anxiety, but he felt helpless and unable to do anything about his problems. In his case I was hoping that we might get a 'One-session Wonder', which is where in just one session of therapy we would cure all of his obsessions in one fell swoop (all therapists get these one-session cures occasionally, and it's great when we do, but the problem is that people then think that you're Jesus!). He told me that when he was a child the family home was broken into by burglars one night when everyone was asleep in bed. They came down the next morning to find that many things had been stolen and also that his pet rabbits had been killed by the robbers. There was a possibility that this traumatic event had caused his obsessional behaviours, so we spent our first session doing EFT (Emotional

Freedom Technique) on this memory. It contained a lot of fear and anxiety, as he relived the child part of him realising their house was not the safe place he thought it was, and that they could have been murdered in their beds. At the end of an hour's tapping he felt great relief, was much calmer and was able to think about that memory without any apprehension.

John returned a couple of weeks later and was able to report that the tapping had indeed had a significant impact on his OCD; he was no longer checking locks and windows on a night before bedtime, and he was not even worried about it anymore. However, he still had most of the other rituals and obsessions still in place. Bang went my hope of a one session cure, and my Jesus delusion took something of a dent, but I realised that this meant that we had more to do to release his OCD. Once in trance in this second session John's IMR signal indicated that the emotional causes of his obsessions were coming from five previous lives. I could see his eyebrow rise quizzically as this signal took place (he told me afterwards that he didn't believe in past lives) but he allowed himself to move into the first past life and soon he was reporting what he was seeing:

> *I'm outside and on a tropical island. I'm a young man with dark skin and I'm wearing a sort of rag around my waist. I'm in the trees, looking at a path to the beach and the sea. I feel good; my wife comes out of the bushes holding our little girl and she's smiling. She has three marks on her forehead; they're like dots that have been stuck on there. Her hair is a long, braided ponytail. We go to a village and my little boy runs up to me and I pat his head. I meet up with about eight other men and we've all got sticks; we're going hunting. We go into the trees and walk for some time but we don't find anything. Suddenly we're attacked; there are rocks and sharpened sticks being thrown at us through the bushes. We run forward but lots of other men come out around us. We run away through*

the trees but we get separated. I'm hiding in thick bush as some of the other tribe run past. One man stops and stands and I run out from where I'm hiding and hit him with a rock on the back of his head. The others hear his cry and turn and run after me. As I run down a path I see two of my people hiding in a ditch but they tell me to keep running. I jump into a ditch and hide. Eventually the other tribe leave and I walk back to the beach and then on to my village. There's no-one around. My little boy has been hiding and he runs up to me and points towards our hut; the baby's dead but my wife's not there. She's been taken. I pick up my son and hug him; I'm crying inside but not on the outside. I feel angry; they'd tried to take my wife before this but we fought them off. Others come out and are looking around, helpless. I just sit with my little boy; he's still crying.

John stopped talking and settled back into relaxation again. I asked him to move to the next significant event in that lifetime. After a few seconds he continued:

It's a few years later and I'm with another man, my best friend, hiding behind trees and bushes looking down into a big village. We're used to fighting. I've told my little boy to go back; he's 13 now. I'm looking for my wife and I see her carrying wood. A big man grabs her and throws her to the ground. She's picking up the wood. She's just a slave to them. We tunnel through the bushes to the village and kill the two guards. I whistle to my wife and she sees me and smiles, but a man sees her smile and then he sees me. Men of the village attack us and they push me to the ground and then drag me to my feet. They tie my wife to a tree; they've found my boy and drag him by his hair. They've tied him there too. I feel angry and helpless. They set fire to wood under them and set them both alight; I'm on my knees and they're making me watch. I'm crying. Then two of the men push a long, sharp stick under my ribs right through me. I'm dying. It's all quiet now.

John relaxed again and I brought him out of trance. He was surprised at how vivid the images were, and even more surprised that he'd experienced a previous life. He was also a little sceptical as to how this would help him with his obsessions, but happy to go through the process to see if it could help him to change.

He came for his next session a few weeks later, telling me that he felt safer and less anxious in himself than he'd felt for some time, but most of the rituals were still firmly in place. I reassured him that this was quite normal, as usually what happens as we go through the regression process is that the problem we are working on gets weaker as we continue to release the emotional causes. Once all the causes have been neutralised then the problem, like Monty Python's dead parrot, 'has ceased to be'.

I took him into hypnosis and guided him back into another past life. This time he was a soldier in the time of war, wearing a dark grey uniform. He looked very tense as he told me what was happening:

I'm in charge of three other soldiers and we're walking into a village. There are houses on either side and it's real quiet. We're holding rifles in front of us and I feel very anxious; it's as if I don't know what I'm doing. The two others say they have to go back and they put me in charge of eight soldiers before they go off in a truck. It feels too quiet to go forward so we go around the village. We go towards a big church where I see more of our men crouched down behind a wall. We're reinforcements for them. Over the hill, in another village close by there's a big fight going on. I feel even more nervous, as if I'm too young to be in charge and I don't know what I'm doing. We run down the road to the other village to where four of our men are behind a wall. They ask me what to do. I send two men into the field to act as snipers but one of them gets shot in the head. We go to the left to where the main battle's taking place and then it all happens so fast. Two men jump out and start shooting at us; we've got nowhere to go so we run down an alleyway. There are only three of us left and we run into an empty house. One of us gets shot as we reach the house. I'm terrified, I feel as if I'm going to die. I just curl up into a ball in a bedroom. I'm so scared I'm almost crying. I stand up in front of the window and get shot in the shoulder. I don't know what to do. We go back down the stairs and run back down the alleyway. We hide behind a big wooden thing and the other man is telling me to shoot to give him cover. He runs out but I can't shoot and he gets shot in the head. I run back up the hill and manage to get away. I sit behind a tree with my head on my knees, crying. I feel ashamed; I blame myself for getting the others killed. Later on I get sent back home and I meet the wife of one of the men who got killed. She says to me that I'd said that he'd be alright with me. I just walk away feeling so guilty. I feel really strange.

Although John was not crying or reacting as strongly as many of my clients do as they experience traumas, his whole demeanour as he relived the past life was extremely serious and his voice had been shaking throughout. He relaxed again though and breathed heavily for a few seconds before he told me that he'd moved onto another life. Once more he became tense as he described being at sea in the engine room of a ship that had a burst pipe that was letting in water. As he tried to fix the pipe with another man, the water rose higher and higher until they were trapped and unable to get out. After feeling panicky for some time he drowned as the engine room filled with water and the hatch to the rest of the ship was under water and so wouldn't open. Having died in that life he felt calm again and he surfaced out of trance feeling peaceful. He told me that he'd always had a fear of water, and it could be that the past life was the main cause of it.

John came back a couple of months later for his final session and he told me that there'd been a big improvement in his fears and rituals. He was no longer doing most of the rituals and he felt that the OCD was much weaker than it had ever been. He still had an issue with the need to hold up door handles though, and the number three was still bothering him. He estimated that he was 80% better, and he felt much more confident too. He had started the new job at the prison and was enjoying his new-found sense of freedom. I knew that we had a bit more to do to get him totally free, and in this final regression session we worked through and released the last two past lives. In the first one he found himself in Russia, wearing thick clothes as a man in his twenties:

> *I'm outside in a village square at sunset with five other men. They're all wearing furs and have beards and fur hats. We've got really old guns. I feel that I'm new to their group and I'm learning things. We go to a man's house who they say was one of their group but he's been taking stuff from them. They're laughing; I don't think we're good people. We walk into his house and he's got three young children; they're saying that he's taken more than he's supposed to. They've shot him! I'm shocked and I step back into a corner of the room. His children run in and the men turn on me, telling me to shoot the kids. I can't and I say it's gone too far. They point their rifles at me and I shoot the main man but they shoot me. I'm laid on the floor dying. They shoot the three children, one by one. I can't move; they shoot me again as they leave. There's no more.*

John was quiet for a time, and then he told me that he was in another life. This time he was a little 6-year-old boy playing with his older sister in a big garden of a big country house:

> *My sister's about 10 years old and she's telling me off for picking an apple; we're not allowed. We go inside the house, there's lots of wooden panelling and mum tells my sister off for getting me muddy. I have to go and get changed. I go back into mum's room and she's crying but she says that nothing's*

> *wrong and she tells us to go away. I feel confused. We go back into my room and my sister tells me what we're going to do. We go down the hall and shout that we're going outside, but we double back and hide behind a big wardrobe. Mum goes out of her room and we sneak in and hide behind some curtains. Mum comes back in and she's packing stuff into a big trunk and dad's coming up the stairs. They start to argue and mum says that she's leaving. He grabs hold of her, pulls her to the floor and starts to strangle her. My sister shouts "stop it" and we run out of the room and into another room and we lock the door. My sister's crying. Dad's shouting to us to open the door; he says that they were playing. My sister's screaming and holding me. He kicks the door open and pulls us off the floor. Mum runs in with a knife and stabs him in the back. He falls and she grabs us and drags us down the stairs. We go outside and there's a carriage waiting; I think she's been having an affair as she runs to the man in the carriage and hugs him. She tells us to get in. Dad's come outside with the knife and he's walking slowly towards us. The man in the carriage pulls out a shotgun and gets out. Mum pulls us in and closes the curtains in the carriage so we can't see. We're crying and mum's hugging us tight. There's a gunshot in the background and the man gets in and we go. That's it, it's gone now.*

This was the subconscious' way of saying that we had finished in that life, so I asked John to come back to full awareness. He was astonished at the totally different nature of both of those lives and he said that although he had felt much fear as he went through them the nature of the fear was different in both cases. He did admit to feeling lighter inside, which is a classic sign that we had released the traumas, and so it proved. I met him a year later and his OCD was totally under control, his confidence was high and he was working in a stressful environment at the prison without any of his former problems.

Chapter 21

Using the Mind to Heal the Body

I love using hypnotherapy to help with physical problems as the results are often dramatic and life-changing for my clients. Pain, for example, is something that regression therapy is very effective at either reducing or neutralising altogether. Getting women pregnant is also something that I have done regularly over the years. Hm ... maybe I'd better rephrase that ... I have helped many women who were unable to conceive by releasing the emotional blocks that were stopping the body from becoming pregnant. I think that sounds better, don't want anyone to get the wrong impression.

Claire was 27 years old when she came to me. She had been trying to get pregnant for some time but had been unable to do so. There were no physical reasons why this was happening (both her and her husband had had medical tests) but she did have a history of emotional imbalances, including a period of anorexia in her teens. This was probably a reaction to her upbringing, which was difficult, as well as a tough time at school where she was bullied. As part of the therapy process we did spend time working on her emotional pain from this life, but there were also several previous lives and some ancestral trauma that needed to be worked through and released too.

It was in our fifth therapy session that we started to move into her past lives, and once she was in trance she flowed nicely into the first of them and began to share with me the images she was seeing in her mind's eye and the feelings in her body:

I'm outdoors, standing alone in a clearing in a wood. I'm a woman; around 30 years old wearing a skirt and a cape with a hood on it and leather shoes that are shaped like slippers. I'm feeling really anxious, as if I'm hiding from something. I see children running out from my house, it's a small hut; I don't want them to see me. I've come out here to give myself some time for myself. I've been crying. The brain I've got doesn't work very fast; as if I'm a bit slow mentally. I've lived here all my life, from when I was little with my parents and my brother. My father got killed but he used to hate me; he was always hitting me round the head and telling me that I'm too pretty and I'm trouble.

Claire looked upset as she spoke, and then she sighed and was silent. I asked her to go to the next significant part of the life and within seconds she continued:

I'm in my hut with a man, sitting on the floor. He's really good looking and I'm attracted to him but he looks out of place as he's smartly dressed. I sleep with him; it's like I'm his mistress. I wish he was kind to me but he doesn't feel anything for me. When he leaves he doesn't acknowledge the children outside. I'm always embarrassed when he's seen leaving my house; the village looks down on me, it's as though I'm the local whore. I hate myself and I punish myself by sleeping with lots of men. I do it for food but I also like it. They often bring watered down red wine and all sorts of basic food. I don't care about my children; I had them with someone else a long time ago. I feel that I've blocked myself from feeling my emotions. I keep thinking about having sex with this man, we have a connection but he won't acknowledge it. It really hurts. I feel really sad and anxious.

Claire began to weep and clench her hands into fists as she continued:

I'm having sex with him and he's on top of me. I have some weird conflicting feelings inside me. I feel dread and anxiety and I don't want to be there but I'm enjoying it physically. There's pain in my stomach from the anxiety. Because he doesn't love me, I feel really angry, it's as though I want to hurt him. I can't stop thinking about hurting him. I relish the thought of beating him up and I have an awful desire to peel the skin off his face with a knife. It feels good to think about putting my hands round his neck and strangling him. When he's finished, I push him off me and he just lies there. I sit in the corner rocking myself for comfort. I feel so anxious but also numb. The scene's fading now; I think I sit in the same corner for hours at a time. It's so sad. It's more distant now.

There was no more for Claire to experience from that life so we did some work to release the emotional pain that she was feeling, including going through the death in that life from an illness in her late 30s. She came out of hypnosis and told me that she felt that the man in that lifetime who she was attracted to but who was just using her for sex was her husband in this present lifetime.

In her next past life Claire was a member of a tribe that was out hunting when she was shot in the neck by an arrow and died. She realised that she had been betrayed by her brother in that life; he it was who had shot her. However, it was her next past life that had a much stronger effect on her. In this she was a young woman living somewhere in Europe during WWII:

I'm a young woman and it's night-time in a city. There are streetlights and it's raining. I'm hiding against a brick wall; I've been running away from some people and I feel relieved that I got away. I feel anxious but as it's a constant feeling I've got used to it; the war has made me feel unsafe. I'm remembering the last time I felt safe was on a family holiday; I'm picturing sitting on a cliff and then going to a chalet in the mountains covered in thick mountain mist. It's cold outside but nice to go inside to get warm. I'm connecting the cold and the wooden chalet to something terrible; I've been taken away to a camp by the Nazis. There's mud and dust and lots of outside areas and I feel incredibly cold. I'm in a wooden hut and it's freezing outside and inside; I'm thinking back to the warm clothes I had on holiday in the mountains because I don't have any here. I feel helpless and can't believe that I can survive the cold. I'd heard rumours about these places before I got here. Older people around me keep dying but I feel quite strong and a part of me enjoys seeing what my body can take. I spend a lot of time, sometimes hours, sitting on my wooden slatted bunk looking out at the open countryside outside the camp. There are loads of people around and so much fear everywhere; if I feel it I think I'll die so I keep my feelings buried. I miss my family and I'm sad that the last time I saw my younger brother we had a fight. Now I don't know where he is. I can't believe that I'm in this place; I come from a big house and a comfortable lifestyle. I feel sad and powerless and I know there are lots of people dying here. There are just a few of us here who have lasted so long. I don't talk to anyone though.

Claire paused at this point as she appeared to move on in time. Her delivery of the experience continued in a monotone voice, as if she was in some way both physically alive but also lifeless and emotionally empty:

The war's come to an end and we're waiting to be rescued. I feel relieved but sad at the same time. The hut is safe and I feel petrified of going back to the outside world. I feel strange about the fact that I'm going to live as I've got used to the idea of dying here. I feel a big feeling of loss because I think my family have all died. As we are driven away in a truck I'm looking back at the camp and feel overwhelmed that it's the first time I've seen it from the outside. I see the first word over the gate to the camp — it's "Arbeit". I feel insecure leaving it as all the structure has now gone that kept me going. Even though everyone's happy I feel alone. Later on I move to America and live an ordinary life. I marry a nice American but I can't love him because I don't know how to and he doesn't know the real me that I keep hidden. I have children but my family don't really know me. I regret that I left the real me back in the camp and since then I haven't really lived. I die quite young, in my 40s. I become ill and after an initial panic I accept it, just as I used to do in the camp. As I'm dying, I realise that shutting down my feelings and not letting anyone in has alienated me, it hasn't protected me. Facing death shouldn't stop you from living.

Claire became quiet and breathed heavily. The life had evaporated from her mental picture screen and she came out of hypnosis. She now had a new awareness that pushing down her emotions is not the best way to approach life, and she reflected on how much she had done so throughout her present life. Whereas in the past life she was, of course, in 'survival mode' all of the time as she could have died at any moment, her present life was completely the opposite, and so therefore it was perfectly OK for her to give herself permission to feel the emotions that she kept bottled up on a day-to-day basis. This new understanding would allow her to start letting go of the locked-in energies that were stopping her from conceiving. Remember, the regression model is that all of our issues come from locked-in feelings and emotions; when we allow our body or our energy field to release them, our issues are released too.

As an aside, Claire was deeply shocked when I told her that the word 'Arbeit' was written on a plaque above the front gate of Auschwitz and other concentration camps for people to see as they entered the camp; it read 'Arbeit macht frei' (which means 'work sets you free').

Claire's next past life in her next session was also filled with suppressed feelings, this time of a sexual nature. She saw herself as a well-dressed, upper-class man in a Victorian-type living room, holding the white-gloved hand of a woman. She put her hand to her head, as if in pain, and spoke through a clenched jaw:

> *I have pain in my head and tension, as if I've just been crying. I'm scared. She's sitting and I'm standing. I've been visiting her and I've told her my secret. I feel stupid in her company but I'm attracted to her in a strange way, but it's not a sexual attraction. She has a power over me; I'm not attracted to women at all but I am to her. She's wanted to have me around her; I think that she finds me useful in some way. Now she knows my secret she's saying that she has the power to tell anyone that I'm a homosexual. A few days later we have a conversation walking along a seafront promenade and she proposes to me, saying that we should get married to protect each other. I don't have any options as she'll tell everyone if I don't. We get married but it's only a marriage on paper and she's used me to get a rich husband. We live together in a bigger house but she's awful to live with and she's having a go at me all of the time. She has the power to do that because I can't upset her too much. I feel like I've given up and the strain of it starts to tell on me; I'm only 40 but I look 60. All the time though I'm still slightly mesmerised by her. One day I just keel over and die, maybe from a heart attack, and even then, she's really cross with me and not upset at all.*

The life was over, with all of its stresses and strains, and the desperate need to hide one's sexuality from a society that abhorred (and treated as criminal) homosexuality in a man.

Once more she had been forced to suppress her emotions in order to survive. Claire started to relax and then she moved into another life, again just as unusual as the others:

> *I'm a man, in some sort of temple in the jungle. It's a secretive place and I'm dressed up in ceremonial clothes and there are other men — the leaders — wearing headdresses. I can smell that we're burning something. I come here a lot but I don't feel comfortable. I feel sick, as if I'm afraid. I'm afraid for my young son who's here too. I feel that I can do something magical but I'm refusing to do it and they're threatening that something will happen to my son if I don't. I feel that I have an enormous connection to the Universe which is normal to me but not to everyone else. I'm like an energy transmitter; I can lift it out of the air and transmit it to others and the bad people make me give it to them so they have power and control over people. It's as if I'm an oracle or a channel and they make me give them knowledge and power. I want to be away from them but I know something horrible will happen to my son if I don't give them what they want. A big chill has just swamped me — I realise that the only way to stop it is to kill myself. My son doesn't have the gift so he'll be OK. They're corrupt and cruel and the only way to stop them is if I wasn't here. I wait for nightfall and I'm sad as I leave my family but I can't tell them. I go to the clearing around the temple and set fire to brush torches as I want them to find me before my body decays in the heat. I take a hallucinogenic drug that I use for ceremonies and then I take poison so I won't feel the agony of dying. I sit cross-legged and as I die, I feel myself floating upwards, feeling sad at leaving behind my family. I feel peaceful now.*

Claire came back to conscious awareness feeling very calm. She couldn't understand how these past lives were connected to her problem, but I guessed that part of it was because her body had been carrying in it an energy of homosexuality, as if her body was confused sexually and the conflict inside her was stopping her from conceiving. Also, it may have been that because of the second life her subconscious was scared to have a child in case something bad happened to them (because of the threats to her son in that life). We discussed things for a while at the end of the session and then she left, hoping that our work was getting her closer to her goal of starting a family.

In her next session, Claire experienced the last of the past lives, although firstly we had to clear some ancestral traumas. In one of them, she relived some painful events that had happened to one of her great-great-great-grandfathers, five generations ago. In this his sons left him to emigrate to America and he felt deep sadness that he would never see them again. This had set up a belief in her own subconscious that if you have children, they will hurt you by going away. In the other she experienced her mother's sadness at only being able to have one child. We can see that again the subconscious was creating a connection between children and emotional pain. The subconscious is very literal; because of the last past life and these ancestors' lives it was saying that children equal pain and death. One of our therapy maxims is that every behaviour, however negative or bizarre, has a positive intention underneath it. By not allowing Claire to become pregnant the positive intention behind it was to protect her from the same misfortunes. It may seem illogical, but the subconscious has a logic all of its own.

Claire's final past life was quite modern but again contained the theme of the repression of deep emotions leading to unhappiness, as well as the recurring theme of powerlessness. Again, when she went into trance her face became stern as she spoke:

> *It's night-time and I'm alone, walking around the outside of a house. I'm a man in my 30s and I feel unhappy as I wander up*

and down. There are lots of people in the house and a party going on. I felt I needed to get away as I couldn't bear it anymore. I have a headache from holding back my tears. I'm in love with a woman inside the house but it's unrequited. The party is because she's got engaged to someone else. I feel tense and desperate but I'm helpless as I can't do anything. Even though I don't think I actually like women, I've completely fallen for her but it's unspoken. I know that she's with someone else but she doesn't really love him. I go back inside and I'm talking to her. I'm totally infatuated with her. I feel desperation and there's a big ball of anxiety inside me; it's a real strain keeping it covered up. At times when she looks at me it's as if she knows but she doesn't want me to say anything. I feel awful as I have one dance with her and I feel torn between loving her and being near her and not being able to say anything.

A tear dropped down her cheek and her lip was quivering as she felt all of the trapped emotions. She didn't speak for a few minutes as she processed what was happening in that life and moved on in time. Finally, she sighed and spoke with a softer tone in her voice:

I'm much older now, sitting at my desk thinking about her. I feel calmer and although I'm sad I don't feel crushed with anxiety and desperation. I'm reading in the newspaper that she's died. I haven't seen her for many years. I'm OK now; I've got a partner, a man who loves me. My regret is that if I were young now, I wouldn't have to repress all my feelings as society has moved on and it's much looser about these things. I feel much calmer now and wiser.

There was nothing else in that life to experience so I brought Claire out of trance. She felt very peaceful, as if she'd let go of something that had been troubling her for a long time.

Although we had no more regression to do, we still did a few more sessions of hypnotherapy and EFT, continuing to release old patterns and heal emotional imbalances. During that time she had a noticeable feeling of happiness and freedom inside her and it was a few months later that she found out that she was finally pregnant. Nine months later she was the proud mother of twins, a boy and a girl. Her subconscious was at last able to accept some new beliefs: it's safe to have children and that children equal happiness.

Chapter 22
Regression for Allergies

'Speak roughly to your little boy,
And beat him when he sneezes;
He only does it to annoy,
Because he knows it teases.'
Lewis Carroll

One aspect of hypnotherapy that is relatively unknown is how it can be used to cure allergies. There is a fairly effective allergy cure technique used by NLP practitioners, but it doesn't always work and my experience is that if an NLP technique doesn't work it means that the emotion that is causing the problem is too deep and needs to be worked on in regression. It may sound odd to think that an allergy can have emotional causes, but I've often found this to be the case. I had one client in Stavanger, in Norway, who had a very bad pollen allergy; every year during spring and summer she was totally miserable as due to the allergic reaction she spent every day sneezing and wheezing and with her eyes streaming. We found that it was caused by a previous life in which she'd died of starvation. However, the link to the allergy was that as she was dying in the past life, she was desperately trying to stay alive by eating grass. This meant that in her present life her subconscious was connecting grass and pollen with death, and because the subconscious has its own logic, once the pollen came out each year it triggered the pain of the death in the past life, thus causing the allergic reaction. Our sessions were quite dramatic as she spent a lot of the time retching and choking and almost vomiting whilst she was in hypnosis experiencing the death. As a result the allergy was completely eradicated and she was able to start enjoying her summer holidays.

Another client in Oslo in Norway had an allergy to latex. This again was a severe allergy; if she ate in a restaurant where the kitchen staff prepared food using latex gloves, she would be very sick and her body would react as if she'd been poisoned. There were several traumatic death experiences in her past lives causing the allergy and once we had released the fear and other emotions by reliving the deaths, the allergy was eased.

Helen was a nurse in a hospital who had been suffering from allergic rhinitis for over ten years. It was making her life unbearable, especially at work, where coming into contact with the smells of certain chemicals, plastics and cleaning materials would make it worse. Her symptoms included itching in her mouth and throat and on her skin. She sneezed many times each day and she also had nasal congestion, coughing, headache, sore throat, and a constant runny nose. Helen's case was unusual in two ways: firstly, because there was a substantial number of previous lives (15 in total) containing emotional and physical traumas that were causing the allergic rhinitis, as well as some major traumas in her present life; secondly because some of the past lives were animal past lives. I realise that this may make you raise an eyebrow, but it does very occasionally happen that a client will experience a past life as an animal in a regression session. I have to be honest and say that I really don't know if the client is merely imagining a life as an animal as it's hard to tell if it's real or not; however, if it helps the client to get better, I suppose it doesn't really matter.

I had a client with spider phobia whose past lives included a life as a baby squid! She experienced a lot of fear as she was swimming around in the sea and the target of many bigger fish and aquatic life forms that wanted to eat her for breakfast. She finally felt safe when she found a small cave to hide in at the bottom of the ocean. Unfortunately, the safety didn't last long as she realised that something else was living at the back of the cave and it slowly came forward to tear off one of her tentacles.

She escaped and managed to survive to become an adult squid. Weird, I know, but it helped her to let go of her phobia.

Helen was a fast worker in her regression sessions, in that she would usually go straight into the trauma in a past life, release the emotions from it and then go into another life straight away. This meant that we would work through three or four past lives in one session. Here are a few of them, including her animal lives:

> *I'm a young woman feeling happy, taking in the scenery on a summer's day. I see trees and greenery and a brook running close by. Suddenly I feel scared as I hear people in the village shouting "fire". I can hear screaming and I run to see a building on the edge of the village is on fire. I feel terrified; I can smell burning flesh and I know that my child is trapped in the building. People are panicking and trying to put the fire out. My child is brought out covered in burns but she's dead. I sit cradling her in my arms. I feel awful. The picture's clouding over and I'm in another life. I'm an Eskimo girl and I'm cold. I'm squatting on the floor when a polar bear attacks me. I didn't hear it coming. It's clawed me across my face and then it kills me. I feel sad as I don't feel ready to die. I'm floating away and now I can see a castle. I'm a man in medieval times carrying arrows on my back. I'm terrified, running away from men galloping on horses after me. Two of them ride on either side of me and the men pick me up and carry me and then drop me under the horses' hooves. They're laughing as they do this and the horses gallop over me and then come back and trample me as I lay on the ground. I'm in agony; the pain's excruciating. It feels like they've broken every bone in my body. They ride off and leave me. I try to crawl to the shade of a tree but I can hardly move. There's blood everywhere and I can taste blood. I've died now and feel peaceful.*

And that was all in her first session! Her second session was just as action-packed:

I'm a young boy, around 5 and I'm terrified. Soldiers are taking my mother away. She's crying and hysterical. I'm confused. They take her away in a cart. I think they're Roman soldiers. I'm sobbing and I chase after the cart but I can't see her anymore. I urinate on myself because of the fear. I think she's been stealing. I won't ever see her again. I run into town searching for her; I ask a soldier where my mother is and he just throws me to the ground. A lady picks me up and asks me what the matter is. She takes me back to her home and looks after me. She says that mother will be kept as a slave now. I'm very sad but she takes care of me. I can't see anymore. Now I'm outside on a warm day in another life. I see trees, hills and corn. I'm a rat and a car's just run over my tail. It's painful and bloody and sticky. I don't feel well and I feel weak and unable to move quickly. A fox attacks me and finishes me off. Now I'm another animal, not sure what type. I'm in shallow water with my mate and a crocodile's attacked me. I'm fighting to escape but it's got my leg and it pulls me under the water and I'm fighting for breath. It's turning over and over in the water until I die. Now I'm in a human life again. I'm a young man, outdoors talking to a man who's sitting on a horse. Suddenly the horse rears up and he falls off and one of its hooves smashes me in the face. I'm in agonising pain. I fall to the floor and there's blood everywhere. The other man's fallen and hit his head on a stone. Blood's pouring from my face and I feel nauseous and sick. I can't get up. Some people come and take me into a village. I try to get up but I keep falling down and the pain in my head is terrible. They lay me in bed and bathe me but I lose consciousness. I think I die from a brain haemorrhage. I've slipped away now and feel calm. It's over.

So, seven former lives (including two animal lives) cleared in two sessions! In our next session Helen began by going into the womb at the start of this present life. Again, this may surprise you but some people experience trauma before birth which stays with them all of their lives and causes problems. I had one client who was massively traumatised when he was in his mother's womb by his alcoholic father trying to abort him by punching his mother in the stomach. As he relived this in trance he was terrified, curled up into a ball with his hands over his head, whimpering and moving from side to side as if he was a tiny baby trying to get away from the blows that were coming at him in the womb. Helen's experience was a little different:

> *I can hear shouting going on outside, there's an argument. It makes me feel anxious. Mum's telling my elder sister off and she's crying. It's all because my father's not her biological father. I feel mum's resentment towards her. Mum's also crying and I hear a thud as my sister slams the door. There's always animosity between them. I feel scared as it's not a calm household to be going into. Now I hear plates crashing as mum's throwing things at my dad. I can feel that she has a lot of anger in her and it makes me upset and fearful. I don't want to be born into this family.*

Having worked through this Helen then moved into another former life:

> *It's medieval times and I'm an elderly woman standing with some others outside in a village. Suddenly men on horseback appear with swords flashing and they're attacking us. People are screaming and dying. I'm cowering, shaking and crying hysterically; I feel so frightened that I've urinated. I can smell death in the air. A man on a horse is coming closer and he thrusts a sword into my chest. There's blood running through*

my fingers and I fall to the ground. I feel my life ebbing away. I don't want to die alone. It's over, my spirit's free now, I'm rising up. I've moved on now and I'm a sparrow sitting in a tree. I'm singing away with lots of my little friends around me. Oh! I see a white cat and it's pinned me to the ground. Its weight's on me, crushing me. I'm shocked and frightened and trying to escape. It's shaking me in its mouth. It's gone quiet now. I've gone into another life. I'm a squirrel in a canopy of trees. I'm busy collecting food for the winter but I see some men below pouring some chemicals into the tree. They're trying to exterminate the squirrels. I'm a lone survivor and I'm scared because there are men all over the place. I've got to hide. Even though I'm hungry I'm too frightened to venture out. I decide to leave this part of the forest and travel to the other side of the woods. I'm cautious but when I get there, I see more squirrels and it feels good to be here. I'm getting images now of an oak tree standing in the middle of a cornfield. I'm in a new life, I'm a nun and there's a storm and I try to shelter under the tree but I get very wet. I get back to the nunnery and I'm in a courtyard with other nuns but I'm very cold and I can't get warm. I change my clothes and they give me some soup but I'm shivering. I get more and more sick. Now I'm in bed, sweating and delirious. I'm feeling weak. Someone's trying to feed me but I'm choking. Eventually I die. I feel shocked.

As you can see, Helen's subconscious simply took her from one life to another in each session. Helen didn't experience a lot of emotion or tension, even though she was aware of the feelings that she'd had in each of the lives, so we were able to move through them quickly and efficiently. In our final session once more she underwent the same process, this time starting in a Victorian workhouse or orphanage finishing with yet another animal past life:

I'm a little child dressed in rags and somebody's beating me. I'm crying with pain and I just want it to stop. I feel as though my bones are breaking. They push me to the floor. Other children help me to get up but I'm wracked with pain. I have to carry on working, folding the laundry. It's hot and my head's bursting. I feel miserable; I'm tired, hungry, thirsty, and my body's very thin. I collapse and they take me to bed, to some straw on the floor. Someone's trying to feed me gruel but I'm too ill to eat. I'm burning up and I just want to die. My life's worthless and nobody loves me or cares about me. I'm getting weaker and then I just die and go into spirit; it's OK to leave as it was a miserable life. Now I can feel a headache and I'm a woman with excruciating pain. It's a migraine and I see flashing lights and I'm sitting being sick. I'm crying with the pain and my mum's getting me some water. She calls the doctor as I've had attacks before but not as bad as this one. My head feels like it's bursting and I'm sitting with my hands on my face and tears pouring down my cheeks. I crumple up onto the floor and start choking, there's lots of mucus coming out of my nose. I feel frightened. The doctor says that I should go to the coast and get some sea air. They pack me off to my auntie's and it has a positive effect on my health. The headaches reduce and I continue to live here happily. I can see the sea. But I've moved into a different life. Someone's throwing a dog over the cliff. I've landed at the bottom of the cliff and I can't move. I'm in so much pain and I'm crying. My owner's a man in Victorian clothes and when his dogs are too old to work, he gets rid of them. I'm in agony and I just want it to end. Someone finds me and they try to pick me up but it hurts so much that I'm howling. They sit with me and stroke me; I feel comforted and I drift off to sleep. I die in peace.

In other sessions we also worked on healing the wounds of her childhood and also neutralising some significant traumas in her later life, as well as some trauma which she had inherited from some ancestors. As a result of all of this therapy she saw a massive improvement in her rhinitis and her allergies. The congestion and other horrible symptoms that she used to suffer every minute of the day were at least 98% better. Maybe the animal past lives were real after all?

Chapter 23
My Spiritual Background

'Your task is not to seek for love,
but merely to seek and find
All the barriers within yourself
that you have built against it.'
Rumi

Writing this chapter is a slightly tricky one for me, because although I realise that past life regression is regarded by most people as a spiritual process, I see it as simply an extension of the regression model and therefore as it's simply a part of a psychotherapeutic process it is not especially spiritual at all. I've said for many years that because Past Life Therapy is such an effective healing modality that it shouldn't be viewed with scepticism by the mainstream therapy community, but should be investigated with an open, analytical, scientific and enquiring mind. If this were to happen, I believe it would gain more credence and acceptance in the therapy world.

Having said all of that, I do realise that in another way Past Life Therapy is a spiritual process because it involves the belief that there is more to life and the world than the physical, mundane 'reality' which we fixate upon every day of our existence as human beings. The idea that we are in some way incorporeal, that we do not simply cease to exist but that our soul continues on a journey after death and is reborn is obviously a spiritual belief (based, I would say, on masses of substantial evidence). The shamanic phrase of 'non-ordinary reality' I think sums up this way of having the mind-frame that everything has spirit (or a soul) and that our soul is eternal.

I'm very lucky in that I class my work as a regression therapist as part of my spiritual path, which means that helping my clients to improve their lives and heal from an array of issues that stop them from living life freely is my way of aiming to make a difference in the world. This I view as a spiritual process, in that serving others acknowledges the universal truth that everything is connected and nothing is separate – we are all one. I work almost every day in past lifetimes, and I am so wrapped up in the concept of death and rebirth that I am sometimes shocked when I meet people who don't believe in the reality of reincarnation.

I expect that like many people, my spiritual journey has been a somewhat convoluted one. I rejected Christianity in my teens (even though I studied Religious Knowledge at grammar school to 'A' Level) and it was when I first read about reincarnation that life on earth finally made sense to me. I was immediately drawn to Buddhism and in my early 30s I started to attend a local group and became a practising Buddhist, also introducing meditation into my daily routine. I didn't think meditating had made much of a difference to how I felt, until one day my wife told me that she had seen a big change in me – 'you're so much less angry than you used to be' were her words. I realised she was right as I had become less reactive to life events that used to trigger me. As I became more serious in my practice and took Refuge Vows, I could feel my levels of compassion opening up too. To take or go for refuge in the three jewels, the Buddha, Dharma, and Sangha, is to make a formal commitment to actualise the Buddha's teachings and path; a commitment to one's own awakening. I studied Buddha's teachings, went on Buddhist retreats and helped to run a local group. After several years though, I became disillusioned with the type of Buddhism I was involved with, which was Tibetan Buddhism. It felt too religious and magical, full of rituals and praying to deities (as it had grown through the early Bon religion of Tibet it had absorbed much of the primitive elements of Bon within its structure).

I left it behind (though I continue to this day to feel strong ties to Tibet and its people) but continued as a non-denominational Buddhist for several years until the reliving of one of my previous lives as a Native American drew me away from Buddhism and into training in Native American shamanism. I liked the connection with Mother Earth, the emphasis on personal development and the sacredness in all things. We were taught that the shamanic training we were undergoing was a warrior path and we had to push through personal discomforts to heal hidden parts of ourselves and to become more balanced. I took part in ceremonies in nature, vision quests, rituals involving drumming and chanting and in many sweat lodges. In the ceremonies I connected with trees (did you know when you're hugging some trees that they exude a latent sexual energy?) and with 'the stone people' and one of the most intense things I did was to spend a night in my own grave! The aim of this ceremony was to 'Make an Ally of Death' and in the middle of the countryside on a remote English farm I spent a full day digging my own grave, 6 feet (2 metres) deep and long enough for me to lay down in. The hole was then covered with boards and a tarpaulin leaving a small hole at one end as an entrance. The earth from the hole was then piled up onto the boards. After smudging and doing a small ritual around a campfire at dusk I was escorted to my grave by the facilitators of the ceremony and, once I had dropped down into it, the hole was covered with boards and the tarpaulin, leaving a small amount of space for air to enter.

As they left, I sat in the grave, in total darkness, feeling very apprehensive. Actually, if I'm honest, I was quite scared. Here I was, in the middle of nowhere, enclosed in a deep hole in the ground until dawn the next morning. As I reflected on the strangeness of my situation (not the sort of thing you can chat about with your mates down at the pub!) I felt very alone. I had a ceremony to complete whilst I was in the grave that would take several hours, and once I had lit a candle and started the process, I began to breathe a little easier as I started to concentrate on the task in hand. Once I settled into my work, I was surprised how comfortable it felt sitting in the grave. It was very peaceful and I felt as if I was being held or cradled by Mother Earth. Eventually I'd finished my ritual and I guess by that time it was probably around 3 a.m. I lay back and rested my head on the earth but as I did so I tuned into my body and my intuition said that there was something else I had to do to complete things. I closed my eyes and drifted into trance (as any normal person would do at three o'clock in the morning in a grave!) and felt myself regressing back into a past life. It was a past life as a Native American medicine man and I relived the death in that life in which I was fighting in a battle and someone came up behind me and tomahawked me in the back (I'd had shoulder pain there for years in this present lifetime). Once I had passed through the death into Spirit, I felt calm and that my overnight ceremony was now complete. However, there was more weirdness yet to come! I spent the next hour or so relaxing and it was then that I began to hear voices singing and chanting. At this stage I wondered if I was starting to go mad, until I realised that it was the facilitators drumming and chanting as they slowly got closer to my grave. The sounds grew louder until they stood above me singing and drumming gently. I felt extremely peaceful and nurtured, both by Mother Earth around me and the kindness of the people above. I was in an altered state of consciousness as I lay there, and then suddenly without warning my upper body swiftly arched upwards and with a jerk I felt something leave my body out of my left shoulder and I flopped back down again onto the floor of the grave. 'What the hell was that?' I wondered as I lay there in amazement.

Then the answer came to me — it was a spirit attachment being released from my body. I didn't know I had one but as they can sometimes hook into our energy fields without us knowing, it didn't surprise me. A combination of the spiritual ceremony I'd undertaken, the reliving the past life and the chanting and drumming above me by a group of spiritual teachers was enough to release it. As the sounds from above moved away and I was left in silence again, I drifted into a gentle trance for a couple of hours. At dawn I was allowed to leave the grave and debrief to complete the ceremony. It was a night to remember in some very unusual ways!

Despite some other intense experiences, after a few years I felt that there wasn't enough emphasis on compassion so I left the shamanic training and for a couple of decades had no spiritual path to follow, other than doing my best to work with my heart with clients in my therapy practice and to live a life centred around kindness. It seems that I was always looking for something that combined compassion for oneself and others, simplicity and a reduction of the ego. I was always repelled by anything that felt too 'religious'. I toyed with Zen and Daoism but I realise now that at that time I didn't truly understand them.

It was in 2020 that a major trauma happened in my life and as a result of a chain of events (which I now understand were meant to happen) I was fired head-first into Non-Duality teachings and, finally, I knew that I had come 'home'. It was as if the scales had fallen from my eyes and the Zen Sutras of Sosan finally stopped being gobbledygook and made total sense (I had been given a copy of these many years earlier but not understood them). Since then my spiritual process has been to focus on being Aware and in One-ness, and thanks to the wonderful Non-Duality teachings of Rupert Spira, my way of being in the world has fundamentally changed and I have more peace in me than at any time in my life. The simplicity of being in One-ness and accepting that everything simply is, has allowed me to be less ego-centred and more in my heart.

Because of this, in some intangible way that I find hard to quantify, my therapy work has deepened and the regressions I have with clients seem to be operating at a deeper level than before. They also go more smoothly; I would guess because I am much more able to hold the space from a place of Conscious Presence for my clients in their sessions.

I am conscious of the importance of therapy to the wider world. As my clients heal from their emotional and physical issues and become more balanced they send out a different energy into the world. They become less reactive and live in the world in a more peaceful state; as they send out this peaceful, more balanced energy into the collective unconscious the world becomes a more balanced place for us all to live in. I feel privileged to be part of this energetic healing of the planet.

Chapter 24
Regression and Relationships

'Men play at love in order to get sex,
Women play at sex in order to get love.'
Anon

Two of the most important things in the life of most human beings are bringing up children and being in a relationship, and in neither of these things do we get any proper training at all. We raise children and get into relationships and simply make everything up as we go along, usually based on how our parents brought us up and how they were in their relationship. It's something of a recipe for disaster, and accounts to a great degree for the insane state of the world that we all live in.

Fortunately the modern world is changing in these respects, in that a few parents do attend child rearing education courses and some couples do go to couple's therapy sessions together, but these are exceptions rather than the rule. Most people just bumble on as best they can; sometimes getting things right, sometimes screwing up spectacularly. With regards to being in a relationship, the interesting thing is that therapy has a lot to contribute to helping people to live in a more balanced way with their partners.

This is done in a variety of ways. Sometimes an experienced therapist will challenge his or her client to begin to look at their own behaviour with their partner instead of just blaming their partner all of the time. This may mean getting the client to look at the patterns that they have learned from their parents' way of being in relationship and becoming aware that they are playing out those same patterns in their own life. With this new awareness the client can reflect on how both partners are responsible for causing problems, not just one of them. I often like to explain that when we are living with someone, we tend to want everything all our own way most of the time, just like we did in childhood, and when we can't get our own way, we go into 'angry child mode' with our partner. Sometimes it's necessary to compromise and recognise that real life is not all about having our own way; being in a balanced relationship involves compromise.

If I have a male client who's struggling in his relationship, I talk to him about a masculine trait that can destroy a relationship insidiously over time. I call this the 'Top Dog' syndrome; this is when a man insists on making all of the decisions, always wants to be the number one and isn't prepared to respect his wife's opinions as 'he knows best'. Over time, this unconscious squashing of the woman causes her to lose confidence and to love her man less and less. It causes resentment and frustration for the woman who isn't being accepted as an equal. I believe that this 'Top Dog' energy is in most male-female relationships and is a hidden cause of damage between couples. To quote the actor Dustin Hoffman when asked about the secret to his long-term marriage, he said: 'I believe that men are selfish pricks and we are not as sensitive, as caring, as nurturing, as women'. The implication being that in order for a relationship to work the man has to become less selfish, less wanting to have his own way all of the time, less desire to be using his 'Top Dog' power. I think Dustin Hoffman has also said that when you let the woman run the relationship (i.e. for the man to get out of his 'Top Dog' way of thinking) then everything runs very smoothly.

I have regularly worked with women who have been squashed in this way for years, and who come for therapy lacking self-esteem and self-worth. This is especially the case if the woman is in relationship with a psychopath male, which is a terrible place for any woman to be. Therapy can help the woman to get stronger and to feel confident enough to make a balanced decision if she should leave the psychopath, and to have the courage to do so. It can also make her strong enough to stand up to an overbearing partner and to start taking her power back.

This is done in a variety of ways, sometimes by using standard hypnotherapy methods, for example using hypnotic suggestions to re-programme her mind so that she feels stronger; sometimes by using NLP techniques to allow her to feel less 'triggered' by her partner. I regularly use Inner Child therapy to help a person to heal and to grow. However, surprisingly regression can also play a big part in helping someone to overcome relationship problems. The main reason for this is that the seeds of a difficult relationship are usually found in the past. These 'seeds' or emotional causes can be the traumas that we carry from this present lifetime, that we bring with us as part of our emotional baggage into any close relationship. When two people get together, they both bring with them emotional imbalances and hurts from the past (often childhood, but sometimes traumas from previous relationships) which sooner or later start to rear their ugly head and can make the relationship go toxic.

They also bring with them events and traumas from past lives, usually with the same person who they are in love with now because that person was around them in previous lives. They also bring with them traumas and relationship pain from their ancestors' lives. All of these things are churning around in the subconscious mind ready to be triggered once we get close to someone. In some cases past lives can bring us closer and reconnect us to someone who we loved in a former life, which helps the relationship to work really well; in other cases the 'unfinished business' from the past lives causes mayhem in the relationship without either partner knowing why.

My sessions with my client, Pete, highlight just how much a dysfunctional childhood can impact on a relationship in adult life. In his early 40s, Pete told me that he was insanely jealous when he was with a woman. He felt paranoid if she was looking at other men and even if she had an innocent conversation in a shop with the shopkeeper, Pete would accuse her of having an affair, wanting to have sex with the man etc. His paranoia would be festering under the surface all of the time and would cause him to have a weekly 'blow out' in which he would become uncontrollably angry and aggressive. He would 'kick off' (his words) and scream and shout at his partner and accuse her of all sorts of betrayals. His first wife had recently divorced him as she couldn't take any more of this, although to rub salt in the wound she had actually had an affair which caused the final break-up of the marriage. Pete had even been imprisoned for a time because of his response to his wife's affair, as he had made death threats towards her new man. His new partner, Sally, was now on the receiving end of his jealousy and was already growing tired of it.

His childhood was awful; his father was a sailor and a violent alcoholic who, when home from sea, would regularly get drunk and wreck the home and beat up Pete's mum. His mother would sleep around with other men whilst his father was away; Pete walked in to find her having sex with another man when he was just a boy. His mum divorced but his stepdad was a nasty piece of work who, every Sunday for six years, would make Pete and his brother fight each other until they drew blood.

We did a couple of sessions of regression into childhood to start the process of releasing some of his anger, fear and sadness that his Inner Child was obviously feeling; as he worked through some difficult memories, he felt very tense and at the end of each session he imagined hugging his Inner Child, giving him love and telling him that he was safe. This problem of not feeling safe is a fundamental part of the human condition; most people do not feel safe most of the time and for many of us the roots of this are in childhood. Pete had rarely felt safe as a child and this had stayed with him into adulthood and was pervading, like a hidden poison, every part of his life as an adult. How our Inner Child feels is how we feel as an adult. If our Inner Child is feeling hurt, frightened and sad, that is how we respond to the world as an adult.

As a result of these sessions, Pete immediately felt better in himself, less anxious about losing Sally and calmer than he had ever felt before. However, he was not fully healed and during those first two sessions he told me that Sally's boss was triggering his jealousy. This was because Sally had told Pete about the way that her boss acted when he was around her at work. He would make sexist comments in the office, which were obviously inappropriate, and also flirt with Sally in a joking way but with an air of seductiveness at the same time. Pete was annoyed by this but was doing his best to let it go. However, when he arrived for our third session, he stormed into my office full of rage. At the office party the night before Sally's boss had gone too far with his seductive comments and after a few drinks had made some lewd suggestions to her and patted her on her backside. Sally told Pete about this at breakfast that morning and he had gone berserk. He told her that he was going to come to her office and that he was so angry that he would kill him and he didn't care about the consequences. He had stormed off but he knew that he had a session with me that morning. Angrily he informed me that he didn't want to let me down so he had turned up for our session, but he was still violently angry and he was going to go to Sally's office after our session and kill her boss! He was very uptight and his speech was loud, fast and aggressive.

I realised that I had to do something to defuse this anger or I would have to inform the police of the situation. As therapists we have a duty to confidentiality but this duty ends if we feel that there is a chance that our client is in danger or is a danger to others. Under these circumstances we have to inform the relevant authorities. With this at the back of my mind, I began the process of talking down Pete's aggressiveness, firstly by mirroring his anger with my voice and tone and by sympathising with him, then by slowly taking the edge and the speed off my verbal tone so that he started to calm down as he subconsciously matched my gradual calmness. After a while he agreed that it would be OK for him to go into hypnosis and once he was in trance, I talked through some metaphors which told the story of letting go of things that are no longer needed and then guided him once more back into childhood memories. I knew that we needed to take as much of the pressure out of his emotional pressure cooker as we could, so that his irrational anger would be reduced. He relived memories of his father beating up his mum when he was only 3 and the police coming to the house and his father fighting with them too; being locked in his bedroom whilst his mum had sex with other men; walking in to his home to find his stepfather having sex with a woman whilst his mother was in hospital waiting to give birth; the baby dying soon after birth and his mum sobbing in anguish. For the first time in our sessions, as he remembered these brutal memories, he allowed himself to cry. As I have stated before, underneath anger there is always sadness, and now he was giving himself permission to feel all of the sadness from childhood that he had suppressed for many years. He realised too that one of his major issues that he had been reacting to was a sense of helplessness. As a child, he had felt helpless and frustrated that he couldn't stop his mum being beaten up by his father and stepfather and that being powerless was one of the roots of his anger.

Eventually he stopped crying and I asked him how he felt — 'softer' was the word that he used. We did some more work visualising Pete being with his Inner Child, reassuring the little boy part of himself that he was safe now and he was loved. When I asked him to come out of trance, he looked very calm. I wanted to make sure that it was now safe for him to leave me, and he was happy to tell me that the murderous thoughts that were at the forefront of his mind when he walked in to see me had now gone. He gave me his word that he was not going to go and kill Sally's boss; he knew that she was just as upset as he was about the situation and that he should leave it to her to deal with it. I don't know which one of us breathed a bigger sigh of relief!

A good example of how regression therapy helped a woman to grow strong enough to come to terms with the ending of a difficult relationship, as well as to become more balanced emotionally, is that of my Norwegian client, Silje. She came to me with low self-esteem, caused partly by a childhood filled with her dad's anger and partly because of intense bullying at school in her teens. The bullying had taken the form of other girls talking about her behind her back and freezing her out of normal school life. One of the things this did was to knock down her self-worth and her self-belief. When she first came to see me, she still lacked confidence because of the bullying, even thinking that she wasn't good looking; despite the fact that she was one of the most beautiful women I have ever seen in my life. Her marriage had been difficult and rocky for over ten years, with a husband who was manipulative and self-absorbed, yet despite this she still felt that she loved him (even though this was in a desperate way). I realised that if we could build up her self-confidence, she would have a chance of standing in her own power as a woman and lose the neediness that characterised her relationship with her husband. I expected that we would work on healing the wounds that she was carrying from childhood so that her Inner Child felt worthy of love, and this of course we did. But her subconscious also indicated that there were several past lives and ancestors' lives that were causing her issues too.

Once Silje had gone into trance in our first session, her subconscious took us into the lives of two of her ancestors to release feelings of anxiety and worthlessness that she had inherited from them. As she was sharing the memories that were being played out on her mental picture screen, she was emotional and her body was jerking and twitching as it released the locked-in energies. Once she had gone through the traumas from her great grandfather's and her father's lives her subconscious took her into the first of many past lives that we had to work through. I asked her to describe what she was seeing and feeling. She began to look scared as she spoke:

> *I'm sitting outside in a street and there are lots of people walking by. I'm a teenage boy trying to beg for money. Most people don't care and they just walk by but I'm used to that. A policeman hits me in the face and says "go on boy, go home". When I get back my dad is there and he's really angry because I haven't brought much money. He's been drinking and he knocks the chair over and gets his belt. I know what's coming. My sister is watching — better he hits me than her. Another day I'm laying cold, naked and hungry in a shed when I hear lots of shouting outside. The door's ripped open and there he is, he's been drinking. He's kicking me in the stomach and the head. I just lie there; I've given up, I can't take anymore. I feel worthless and ashamed. Then I've gone, I'm dead. He digs a grave in the back yard and buries me. I stay around for a while watching him and then I leave and go up.*

Silje came out of trance and emphasised how worthless she had felt throughout the regressions, feelings that she knew had influenced her greatly throughout her present life. She knew that one of her goals was to build her self-esteem so that she could start to live her life in a more confident manner.

In our next session Silje explored some memories from her marriage in this life, in which her husband had badly let her down before she moved into a past life that connects back to my earlier chapter on the persecution of witches:

I'm a young woman collecting herbs in the woods. I'm alone and I feel happy as I'm going to use the herbs to help someone to give birth. I go to a house in the city and make an herbal potion. It's the woman's house and I'm there as she's giving birth; I know that she's expecting a boy. Something's wrong and the baby's stuck and there's lots of blood. I'm trying to help but the woman's very ill and almost unconscious. I'm trying to get the baby out but I haven't done this before. The baby's going blue but I manage to get it out; it screams but the woman's gone. Her husband comes down and he's angry and saying that I killed her and that I'm a witch. I feel scared and rejected as I did my best. I run to the woods and hide but people come for me and take me into the city. People are yelling and spitting and throwing things at me. They take me to the river and there are lots of people there.

Silje began to cry and her body to shake and jerk uncontrollably. Her breathing was rapid as she continued:

They tie me to a stake — I know they're going to kill me. I can see my father in the crowd; he just stands there. He doesn't do anything; he should be protecting me and keeping me safe. He's just shut himself down. I can smell the smoke as they set fire to the wood beneath me. I'm so scared. It's so hot. I tell myself that I'm never going to trust anyone ever again.

She continued to shake and writhe around in the chair as she went through the death process, before she relaxed and her body softened. I asked her subconscious if her father in that life had been reborn in this present life and it said 'yes'. She told me that she knew that he had been reborn as her husband in this lifetime.

When Silje returned a few weeks later she said that she had done a lot of processing after the session but she still had a lot of anger towards her husband. I guessed that as we had cleared the first past life of its negative effects and she still felt angry, that there were probably other former lives where they had been together which we still had to release. This proved to be the case. In this session, as she moved into another past life, she began to hold her neck as she lay in the chair:

> *I can feel pain in my neck. I'm having my head chopped off. I've done something really bad. I'm a man and I've stolen some gold coins and been caught. My friend betrayed me and told them. They tie my hands behind me and drag me along the ground and throw me in a cellar. There are big rats running around. I know they're going to cut my head off but I'm not too scared. I've had a good life with lots of women and beer. They're coming; I can hear the keys jangling. A fat man drags me outside and there's a crowd there. Now I feel anxious when I see the scaffold. I see my friend there, the traitor. I spit at him, then nod to a woman in the crowd. It's time. I'm kneeling with my head on a wooden block. I see old drops of blood on the ground in front of me. Then "swish". The first blow breaks my neck and the second blow cuts it off. As I go into spirit, I'm annoyed with myself because I should have been a better person and fulfilled my potential. The man who betrayed me is my husband now.*

She relaxed for a few seconds but the mention of her husband triggered something and she told me that she had gone into another lifetime, this time in India as a woman:

> *I feel anxious. I'm quite heavily pregnant. My husband has come home from work and slaps me in the face because I haven't made his dinner. He's yelling at me. I just give up; he's always like this. I sit on the floor in the bedroom and he's still angry and he's punching me in the stomach. He's trying to abort me and I'm screaming and crying. He leaves but later something*

happens. I see him lying on the floor with a knife in his back — I did it. I don't feel sad. I feel free. They take me to prison and I get hung but it doesn't matter because I feel free.

Once more her husband had been with her in that past life. This became a recurring theme in the past lives that we explored in our coming sessions:

I'm a woman and I'm laid outside with a big rock on my chest. There's been an avalanche. I can see my little girl is buried next to me; I see her red coat. I can't move and I'm dying. My husband comes and finds me. He knows I'm dying so he tells me that he knows I'm in love with his brother and I've been having an affair. He knows that our little girl wasn't his. We were on the way to his brother's when the avalanche happened.

She began to cough and move her head:

He's put his hands over my nose and mouth to suffocate me. He's helping me to die.

After a few moments she stopped struggling and she sighed. She was quiet for a while and then she told me that she was in another life:

I'm a woman standing barefoot in the sand. I'm in the desert and I can see white tents around. A little boy runs up to me and takes my hand and pulls me towards the camp. He's dressed in a white gown and a white turban on his head. We sit in the shade outside a tent and eat some fruit. I go to get some water and then hear the sound of horses. I feel scared as I can see lots of sand and dust as they ride into the camp. They're tearing the tents down. I grab the boy and run. A man on a horse chases me

> *and hits me on the back of the head with a sword. I'm lying in the sand, dying. The boy's next to me, dead. His eyes are open. I can't feel anything now, and I'm looking down on the body. I see the man who killed us and feel his regret that he killed us. A long time ago I lived with his people and he was my neighbour. We played and grew up together. Then I was sent away to work for a family and we travelled the desert. He didn't know it was me that he was attacking until it was too late. I know him in this present life — he's my husband.*

Once more Silje was silent and then she told me that she had moved on. She began to cough and gasp for breath. Her body was jerking as she spluttered out the words:

> *I'm lying on a board and I can't breathe. There's water in my mouth and my nose. Someone's holding me down, pressing on my chest. It's a priest. I'm a woman; they think I'm a witch. They're checking if I'm a witch. If I die, I'm not a witch. There's something in my mouth. A man close by is very sad. He wanted to marry me but his family is rich so he's not allowed to marry me. We meet secretly but they find out and accuse me of being a witch. I live alone in my cottage making herbal remedies and they came to get me; I wasn't expecting it. I'm screaming as they take me. They're accusing me and spitting at me and they put me on this board into water. I'm drowning and I'm helpless. I've died and they lay pennies on my eyes. I was only trying to help people and I've been punished for it. The man who loved me is my husband now.*

I continued to have further sessions with Silje, and over time her marriage continued to deteriorate whilst she tried to hold it together. The sessions helped her to remain as balanced as she could be throughout this difficult period, but as before several of them contained past lives in which her and her husband were together in various ways:

> *I'm being hanged and I can feel the pain in my neck. I'm a man, around 30, and there's a group of people watching. They're doing it to cause me as much pain as possible. The tips of my toes are just touching the ground so it's not fast. I feel scared and ashamed. I stole a prize-winning pig because my family were starving. I had no work so I was going to sell it in another town. I got caught on the way there. The pig's owner and some of his men are hanging me. I'm dying now. I'm aware that my wife is my husband in this life.*

In another life she was a little girl who was pushed from a bridge into a river by a bigger boy. She hit her head on a rock and dies. Yes, you've guessed it; her husband was the boy who killed her. Her husband was her husband in another life too:

> *I'm a woman being beaten by my husband. It's a regular event. I feel numb as he's punching me. I just give up; it passes quicker if I just lie there. Afterwards I put on my make-up and pretend to our visitors that everything is alright. When they leave, he's angry and he rapes me. I go to bed crying. I stop eating and get thinner and thinner. Eventually I get sick and die.*

Silje was also having real problems with her stepdaughter, who compounded the difficulties that she was having in the marriage. The girl had never allowed Silje to get close to her and as she got older, she became very quarrelsome towards her, behaviour which her husband rarely challenged. The stepdaughter appeared in several past lives too, in each one of which she was the aggressor towards Silje. Working through these particular lives enabled Silje to get a deeper understanding of why the girl was being so difficult and she became less reactive towards her whenever the girl started to cause trouble. In turn this took some of the energy out of the situation, with her and the stepdaughter becoming less antagonistic.

In another session she was in a past life in which she was a male soldier who had to say goodbye to his family before going off on a suicide mission. His youngest son was Silje's husband in this life. As he lay dying with a spear through him, Silje felt intense sadness and guilt that he would not be there for the boy as he grew up. Her next life was interesting as her husband was the ghost of her dead father:

> *I'm a baby lying in a crib. My mother picks me up and I feel good. But my father is cold and hard and when I think about him, I cry and feel anxious. I don't like him. She lays me down to sleep and leaves me alone but I feel scared and I can't sleep. It's dark in the room and I feel as if he's there. It feels as if someone is watching me but there's no-one there. I cry and my mother comes in and takes me to her bed. I'm a bit older now but it's still happening. I can feel the spirit of my father there in my room. I feel scared all the time. He wasn't alive when I was born. He tried to hurt me when I was in the womb by hitting my mother in the chest very hard and she fell. When it happens, I feel so frightened. She pushes him and he falls down the stairs and dies. He'd hit her a lot before that.*

So, if it wasn't bad enough in that life that he was brutal towards her when he was alive, he continued to cause her fear when he was dead too.

The next life featuring her husband connected to Silje's fears that her husband would die or leave her. In this, she was a twin in the womb but the other foetus (her husband in this life) was miscarried and dies. She spent the rest of that life feeling lonely, as if a part of her was missing. Another life had her and her husband together as husband and wife, but he was cruel to her and would badly beat her.

The way in which Silje and her husband changed roles over many lifetimes was fascinating. Sometimes he was the aggressor towards her; sometimes he was close to her and cared for her. Sometimes she was the male and he was the female. In some lives they would tragically lose each other, as in these two lives which came through in the same session:

> *I'm a woman on the edge of a cliff or a mountain and I'm holding onto the hands of a boy who's hanging off the edge of the cliff. I'm trying to pull him up but it's raining and he's slipping. Our grip is slipping. I slip and he falls. I scream and run, trying to find a way down. I find him at the bottom; he's breathing a little but he dies. I have a terrible pressure in my chest. He was the boy who helped me to watch the sheep in the mountains and after his funeral his father blames me. I feel so guilty and not worthy of being loved or close to anyone after his death. I live alone for the rest of my life. Now I've moved into another body. I'm a soldier in a war and I've been wounded. My chest hurts and I'm lying in a tent which is a field hospital. A female nurse is changing the bandage on my chest — it doesn't look good. I can't breathe. She's holding my hand. She has the same eyes as my husband. She holds my hand as I die.*

One more past life in which she lost him was as a woman who dies in childbirth leaving the baby (her husband) to live on without her. The final life that came through was an unusual one with an interesting narrative, with a strange and spooky ending. As it opened up in her mind she smiled and started to laugh:

I'm a young woman wearing a silky red and yellow corset. I'm lying down and an artist is painting me. I think I've had some wine; I feel frisky. He's handsome, with a moustache that curls up. My hair is big! Someone knocks on the door and soldiers come in with rifles and bayonets. They're looking for something and start going through his drawers. He's trying to charm his way out of it. I lie there observing, drinking more wine. They take him away and I'm left alone. I look at the painting; they've ripped it with a bayonet. I think to myself 'what a shame as I look so good'. I go to a bar. I think I'm a prostitute but I'm not working today so I'm just drinking. I feel pretty good and I'm trying to decide if I want to work tonight after all. I walk up to a man playing the piano in the bar and lean against it and start singing. There are no fun men out this evening so I get bored and go to bed. I sleep well; I think I have a good life. I wake up and smell smoke. The inn is on fire and as I run out of my room the staircase is collapsing in flames. I can't go down so I go back into my room and tie some bedsheets together and I climb down out of a small window. I'm very calm; I have an easy-come easy-go personality. I go to another house and knock on the door and a man opens it and goes white when he sees me. He usually comes to me in the bar but he's married. I ask him if I can stay there and he can't say no. His wife's not happy; she's all red-faced and flushed. He says I can sleep in the servant's chamber and I start demanding things, saying that I need clothes and some brandy to calm my nerves. But I don't have any nerves, I just want brandy. I stay with them for a while and help out around the house. His wife is very angry but I don't care about anything; I just take everything as it comes. They have a teenage daughter and we have so much fun, which annoys his wife even more; I like it that way. Later on I use this man to trick another man that I'm better than I am. He's rich and lives in a mansion. I hide my history from him. I get pregnant to him and have a baby boy but he's a big baby and I lose a lot of blood during the birth. I'm afraid that I'm going to die; it's the first time that I've felt any negative emotion. I'm hovering between life and death and I can see the ghosts of two children, a boy and a girl, looking at me. The boy has his finger over his mouth and is going 'shush'. I'm not in my body and it's all a bit creepy. The ghosts take me into the cellar and they're singing a song — 'there are some secrets you never should tell'. Nothing else happens; they just sing that over and over. As I die, they're still singing it. I'm aware that they're both angry; I think that they were abused in that life and maybe they killed themselves. They were his children from his previous marriage and he and his father were abusing them. They made a suicide pact and died together. My husband's mother knew about it and she disliked me. I can sense that they're still in spirit and are around me in this present lifetime. They want to be sent home and they want their bones to be reburied so they can go home to the light. I need to honour them and their pain. I'm imagining burying their bones in a special place. They're thanking me and now they're leaving this earth plane and going into the light. It's done now and I feel calm.

Silje's fascinating journey through the past lives that connected her to her husband was over. As we were going through our regression sessions her marriage became more and more difficult and eventually she found the courage to tell her husband that she'd had enough and she wanted him to leave. She was obviously very hurt but because of the work we had done, taking the energy out of past lives that were binding them together, she had let go of the desperation that she used to feel about being with him. Her subconscious had allowed her to loosen the chords that were holding them together so that over time she became less and less dependent on him; when the break finally came, she was able to take it in her stride and move on. She now felt much more confident and the neediness that had been a feature of her relationship with him was gone. Even through a messy divorce in which he made things as difficult as possible for her, she remained resolute in her determination to move on with her life. The releasing over time of the past life connections had done the trick and she could now stand in her own power. Afterwards she told me that having these therapy sessions was 'the most important loving thing that I have ever done for myself'.

Chapter 25

Only a Slightly Troublesome Little Cough

'All her hair
In one long yellow string I wound
Three times her little throat around,
And strangled her.'
Robert Browning

One of the vagaries of a therapist's life is the unpredictable nature not only of therapy sessions, which can sometimes go in a totally different and unexpected direction (and which the therapist must be alert to and respond to with the calm assurance of a skilled sailor who changes course when he feels the wind changing), but also the way in which a client's issue may suddenly change in scope during the therapy process. Some clients will come with a specific problem, but once the subconscious starts working on it we find that the presenting problem is not the real issue, but that there is something else underneath which needs to be worked on in order to heal the client. Other times a client will present something which seems relatively insignificant but once we begin to work on it, we find that there is a raging volcano underneath. My next client is an example of the latter.

Kari was a nurse who also had a background in complementary therapies. A very self-aware and spiritual woman with a beautiful energy, she had suffered for 15 years with a constant, tickling cough. There was no medical reason why this would be and she was a non-smoker and fit and healthy in herself. She was also not particularly anxious, which would normally be the case with someone with a nervous cough, but the cough was with her all day every day, whatever she was doing. She did notice tightness in her throat from time to time especially if she was feeling stressed, but apart from that she had no other symptoms. She wondered if the emotional cause of the cough was to do with not speaking out or not being heard, especially as she had recently finished a difficult 14-month relationship with a man who was a psychopath and an alcoholic with violent tendencies. I suspected that this relationship had traumatised her, especially as she had spent a lot of time walking on 'eggshells' around him (something which can lead to Post Traumatic Stress Disorder if it goes on for a long period of time), and I expected that we would need to work on her time with him to release that trauma. However, the cough had started at least 12 years before she met the psychopath, so obviously living with him was not the cause. The real causes were a whole series of past lives, far more than I had expected for a problem which was not life threatening or which was not seriously impairing the quality of her life. Most issues that I meet in my work have anywhere between one and seven previous lives causing them; Kari's cough had over twenty! As well as these we also had to release some ancestral trauma as well as some significant emotional events from this present lifetime.

Kari was a fast worker in our sessions; she went into trance quickly and entered past lives easily. In our first session, once she had accessed trance, she relived some memories of her time with the psychopath. As she did this, she was emotional; her body jerking to release the fear that she was feeling. She then went into four former lives, in each of which the psychopath was the aggressor towards her:

> *He's my brother and it's wartime and he has to leave me so he kills me. I loved him and he cuts my throat with a knife. As children we played together. Suddenly he does it and there's blood on my throat.*

She began to cough as she spoke:

> *I feel betrayed by him. He betrayed me in this present life too. I hate him for what he did. After I die he's crying and he closes my eyes. I feel angry, and the feeling of anger has taken me into another life. He's the captain of a pirate ship and I work on his ship. I'm afraid of him. It's not fair; he makes me walk the plank. I fall in the water and the boat goes off and I drown.*

Again Kari was coughing as she felt the water entering her lungs and the feeling of being unable to breathe. She passed through the death and then relaxed again before she moved into another life:

> *He's my father. I'm his son but I'm not good enough for him, I'm not the tough guy he wanted me to be. He's angry and he says that I'm weak and hopeless like my mother. I grow up with lots of fights; he beats me up and my mother too. I start drinking because I'm so unhappy. I want to kill him but I can't. I try to have a relationship with a woman but she doesn't want me and I hang myself. I can feel the tightness of the rope around my neck as I die. I've moved into a Native American life now and I have to be quiet. My husband tells me that I have to be quiet as he doesn't like my voice. I loved to sing. My father is the chief and my husband wanted power so he married me but he likes other women. I tell my father about it but he hits me and says that this is what men do. My husband hates me so much that I don't like to be around him or have sex with him; he's a brute. He's jealous of me because people like to hear me sing around the fire. I try to run away as I'm afraid of what he might do to me. I'm running through woods and across a river. He's following so I run into a cave to hide but that was stupid as I'm stuck. He finds me and takes me back. He punishes me by cutting my throat. I survive but it damages*

my throat and my voice so I can't sing anymore. I'm crushed; I had freedom and now I'm like a slave again. I just give up. I get older and have children but I have no happiness in my life, even my children don't love me. I remember being a child, in a house playing with my mother. I feel safe but some Native Americans come and attack my mother. She screams and fights but they slit her throat. They burn the house down and take me with them; I ride off on the front of one of the horses with one of them holding me. My father and brother weren't there when they came. They take me and make me into a slave. I miss my mother; I never cried for her. Eventually I die and I'm happy to leave. I can sing again and my mother's spirit is there as I die.

As you can see, in each of the lives there was some sort of assault on the neck or throat which had left an energy of trauma in her energy field. That energy of trauma had been brought into this life and was part of the reason why she had the cough. Kari returned a month later to tell me that after the session the cough had immediately reduced by around 80%, although in the last week it had started to come back again and was now only 60% better. I explained that it was likely that the reason it had started to come back is that her subconscious was already tuning into the stuff we would be working with in this new session and it had started to resonate with the traumas we needed to release. This often happens in regression therapy; the subconscious knows what it wants to work on in each session and several days before the session takes place it is already tuning into the traumas that are going to be regressed into in the session.

Once she was in trance Kari moved into a new past life, one which didn't seem to connect to the psychopath but which again involved trauma to her throat:

There's a war going on and people are going off to fight. I'm a little girl, around 5 or 6 and I feel sad because my father is going off on a train. Maybe I'm a Jew as I can see a star on my clothes. My father was taken away from us. My mother and I are also sent to a concentration camp and I'm scared. I see people being beaten. I'm in a shower with my mother and a lot of other people who are crying. I don't understand what's happening and everyone is scared and no-one cares. Then the gas comes and everyone is coughing.

Kari, at this point was also coughing as she cried and her body jerked as if she was struggling to break free from something. Then she relaxed. *'It's quite quick. After death I stay in spirit for a while as a ghost and then I leave. I'm together with my family again.'*

She was calm again and she looked happy for a short time. However, her face then looked troubled and she started to cough and cry. Her body was shaking uncontrollably as she spoke about a new past life:

I'm the young mother of a little girl. We both have blonde hair and we're in the desert. I feel unsafe, as if there's danger around. I've been travelling with my husband in a wagon but some men on camels stop us. They're touching my blond hair. We've been taken away; my husband gave me and our daughter away to save his own life. It's the psychopath who is my husband. He's betrayed me again. The men take us away but I'm fighting and yelling so they stab me in the stomach. I'm frozen in fear but I'm dying. I was very happy before it happened; I was looking forward to the journey and then it happened. As I'm dying I'm telling myself that I can never be safe and you can't trust life.

She breathed heavily for a while and softened a little, but soon her body became tense again:

I'm still feeling that life can't be trusted. I'm a 5-year-old boy and I'm lying on the ground with my legs pulled up and my arms across my chest. I'm in pain. A group of men have caught me and they're cutting me with knives. There's blood everywhere and I'm in agony. They're enjoying it and they take their time over it. I was walking in a street and it was dark and they jumped out on me. One of the men is the psychopath. I was going to where my mother was working. I'm looking forward to seeing her. Just like in the last life when I was looking forward to the trip and then something bad suddenly happens. As I die Light Beings come to me and they're smiling and they take me away. I feel calm now.

Kari came out of trance and expressed amazement at how many times the psychopath had betrayed her in her previous lives. These past life betrayals compounded the numerous ways that he had betrayed her in her present life and had therefore caused an even bigger impact upon her in the 14 months that they had been together. Without her realising, although we were ostensibly working to release the cough, we were also working to heal the emotional wounds that the psychopath had caused her in their relationship only a couple of years before. However, as we went on with our regression sessions, we found that we were also working on her mistrust of men generally, including her present husband (who she had met and married after she broke up with the psychopath). We continued to release trauma from this present life as well as from the lives of several ancestors, and then in a couple of sessions worked through several past lives and an ancestor's life:

The sun's going down as I'm flying in a small aeroplane, a bi-plane. I'm co-pilot and I feel afraid. We're on a reconnaissance mission during a war and I'm worried that I'll die. I'm shooting as we try to get away from another aeroplane; it's hit us and we lose power and we have to crash land. The pilot is trying to get out of the wreckage but I'm stuck. He looks at me and then runs off in case it blows up. I feel alone and helpless; I'm trapped and can't get out.

Suddenly Kari jumped and then flopped down in the chair.

It's exploded and I'm dead. I'm in spirit but I feel shocked. I'm sad thinking about my wife and children. I've been wondering if the pilot has been having an affair with my wife. I don't trust him as he's a handsome, flirty guy and he likes my wife too much. I don't think he did enough to get me out of the plane so it's a double betrayal. I'd argued about him with my wife before I left and she says that he's just flirting but I feel suspicious. My lack of confidence comes from my childhood, where I was shy and quiet. My father's an alcoholic and he hits me a lot, telling me that he doesn't like noise so I have to be quiet. There's no love in my childhood; it is not a happy home. I feel like I put all of my feelings into a block of ice so that I don't have to feel them. I joined the military so I don't have to feel my feelings; I have to be strong and macho. I think that my father is the psychopath. I remember getting bullied as a child and one of the bullies is my husband now. I don't know why my wife married me; I don't feel good enough. Most of my life I don't want to live. I don't feel that I can trust anyone. I can't show love to my wife. I've been a disappointment as a father and my son feels rejected because I can't give him love. His eyes are the last thing that I see as I die.

Kari started to cough as she re-experienced the death in that life, telling me that it was smoke from the burning aircraft that was causing her to choke. Eventually she stopped coughing and moved into three shorter past life experiences; in one of them she was a woman being badly beaten and killed by her husband, in another she was a man who was betrayed by a friend (who was her husband in this current lifetime) and died in a factory accident, in the last one she was a young girl being suffocated and killed by her alcoholic father (the psychopath from this lifetime).

She then moved into a female ancestor's life, many generations ago:

> *She's a strong woman and I feel angry and sad. I fight but men do whatever they want to do. I feel like I give up. I have a child and my husband wants to send him away to work but I don't want it as he's only 8. I fight but they take him and he goes off on a horse. He's scared but he wants to be a big boy. I'm never the same after this; I feel like I've lost a part of myself. I hate my husband and I don't want to live anymore. I get hard after this and push a lot of anger at my husband; he becomes scared of me. I push my daughter away too and she's scared of me. I can't take it anymore so I go into the barn and hang myself from the roof. My daughter finds me — I didn't think that might happen.*

Throughout all of this Kari was sobbing and jerking and she started to cough when she felt the rope around her neck and her body hanging. At the end of the session she felt exhausted but lighter inside. She knew that she had let go of some deeply held negative emotions.

When she came back for her next session, she said that she had been coughing less and feeling more at ease. Once she was in hypnosis we worked through just one previous life, a life full of suffering and with lots of detail:

> *I'm feeling scared. I'm a black man with chains around my neck and I've been taken away from my family. I know I'll never see them again. I'm in the hold of a big slave ship with lots of others. The smell in here is terrible. I was out hunting when they took me. I fight hard but they knock me unconscious.*

My head's bleeding and my eye is swollen and I can't see out of it. I can taste blood and my face really hurts; they really hit me hard with something. I'm a strong man and I'm angry; they put chains on my wrists and chain me to another man. I ask him if he's ready to run. I kick one of them and we try to run but he keeps falling. I try to fight them as they hold me down and put a chain on my neck but there's too many of them. I thinks it's somewhere on the Ivory Coast. They put me in chains with the others and I know I can't get away, but I still feel proud, they haven't broken me yet. I'm chained up in the ship with others on either side of me; it's a long voyage and we go to other places to pick up more slaves, mainly women and children. How can they survive? There's so much sadness in here. There's not much food and the water stinks. I feel weak and thirsty. People get sick and are throwing up; the stink is awful. I can hear the ocean outside and feel the rocking of the boat. I'm so hungry but the food is just thrown at us in our faces and it tastes bad. My mouth's very dry and sore. I was strong and healthy at first so my face heals. We have to shit and pee where we lay and we lose all dignity. I feel sorry for the children as many of them die. There was a beautiful girl, about 12 years old, who's now just skinny. She cries a lot and calls for her mother. In the beginning they took her out for sex and when she came back she was crying. They are animals and they treat us like this; they're white devils and they're not human. They've destroyed the girl. I hope they didn't take my wife; I think about her a lot. I want to kill them but I feel angry, sad and helpless. I'm so weak now and I just sleep a lot of the time. I expect to die here. After a long time the boat stops and I feel fresh air. They're whipping us to get out but I can't stand on my feet and I fall on the floor into the piss and shit. It hurts to move because I've been lying still for so long. I have to drag myself out and it's good to be outside in the fresh air. We lay on the deck and they throw cold water on us to clean us — oh, that was cold! My legs are stiff and two men hold me and help me to walk off the ship and then throw me to the ground. I crawl to a tree, pull myself up and stand up holding the tree. I want my dignity back; I want to be strong again so I can fight these bastards. They put us in wagons and I'm so tired I fall asleep. They drag me off and put us in a cellar which doesn't smell nice. We're here for some time. I'm surprised I survived. They give us food and water and we can go out sometimes, but not everyone at the same time as they don't want us to escape. I eat and sleep and get stronger but I wonder how my family are. I'm not sure if the young girl on the ship survived, I think she died. I try to run away once but I don't know where to go and they catch me and beat me. My left eye is hurting and I get bitten by their dogs and I get an infection and get sick. I get better though. I'm in a market place now with a chain around my neck and there are lots of people around. Some of them are touching me and feeling my muscles — I think to myself 'you should have seen me before!' They look inside my mouth like I'm some sort of animal. I growl at them so they whip me. I'm sold to a man and taken to a big farm; I think I stay here for the rest of my life and I get a new wife and children. I'm never happy though; this is not my home and I think a lot about my first family. I work in the fields and it's hard work but we grow as a family and although it's hard work it's not the worst place to be. I never try to escape as I don't know where to go and I'm afraid the dogs will bite me. I marry a woman who talks the same language as me and have a son to her and I get some respect from the other Negroes. The whites call us 'niggers' but I'm proud of my people and where I come from. The man who bought me is OK and I just accept this new life and that they killed the warrior in me. I lost a part of myself and I'll always miss my family and my people. I'm quite old when there's an accident and a wagon and a horse fall in the fields onto me; something goes through my stomach and I'm bleeding. My stomach is badly damaged. My son is holding my hand and crying; he's a good boy but this is his country as he was born in America. My heart is in Africa. I say goodbye to him and then she's there — my beautiful wife has come for me. She looks just the same, the same smile and the same eyes. She tells me that our son is still alive. We're looking out over the ocean together.

Kari lay quietly with a gentle smile on her lips, happy that she was reunited with his first wife in spirit and the life was complete. She came out of trance and felt peaceful, as though something had been laid to rest inside her. When she came for her next session the cough had continued to reduce in severity and she said that the past life as the black slave had stayed with her but in a nice way. She felt good feelings coming from it whenever it came to mind.

Once more, in this session Kari went into trance and regressed back into more past lives:

I'm a man and I'm lying on my back on the ground with something round my neck holding me down. A man in a cowboy hat is standing over me; he wants to kill me. I've done something stupid and he's angry. He wants to keep me away from his wife; I've been messing around with her but I was drunk and it was only a bit of fun. He hits me on the side of the head with a spade and leaves me to lie in the sun for a while. He comes back and threatens me that he'll kill me if I don't leave his wife alone. I'm already married with a wife and two children that I love and I'm frightened that I'll lose them if she finds out about this. He tells me that I can stay here overnight and think about what I've done. I feel helpless. I know that he's the psychopath in my life now. Later on some Native Americans find me and start torturing me. I'm shocked that this is happening as I was only having fun when I was drunk. They slit my throat and then spear me and I die.

Kari had looked serious all the way through this and at the end she was coughing as she had her throat cut, but once she died she settled down and relaxed into a deeper trance. Then she became emotional, a signal that she had moved into something else. She continued to cry as she spoke, at times sobbing as she felt the emotional pain:

> *I'm a little girl and I feel sad because people are not nice to me and over time it damages me; I grow up feeling angry and bitter and because I don't like myself I grow up being not nice to others. I'm not nice to my daughter and although in one way it breaks my heart, I can't help it. I run away and leave her when she's 7 because I think it's best for her not to have me in her life. I miss her though and I start drinking so I don't feel the pain and I mess around with men. I want to see her again so I stand outside her school and watch her when she's playing. She doesn't look happy; I wanted her to have a better life but I think she's sad. She sees me and runs to me and she cries and cries and asks why I went away. I tell her that I thought she'd be happier without me. She still loves me and misses me. I messed everything up again. Her father has another woman now so I don't know what to do. I go home and talk with him and he's shocked; he's in love with the other woman. We manage to work something out. I learn from this and stop drinking and I start spending time with my daughter and giving her love. My mother died when I was a little girl and I got the blame for it. I went to live with my father and an aunt and I was in the way and got no love. I was playing in the street with a ball when a car came and I didn't see it. My mother pushed me out of the way and the car hit her and she died. I wasn't allowed to play in the street. My father's shouting at me that it's my fault. I become a difficult child and I disconnect from my heart. I see that bad things can come out of love — my mother's love for me caused her to die. So I close my heart down so nothing bad can happen.*

> *I grow older and get grandchildren and they help me to open my heart. When I'm dying, I thank my daughter for showing me so much love and she kisses my forehead. I just wish I'd showed her more love. I die with a lot of regret and take it with me as I can't let go of it. I spend some time in spirit after I die around her, trying to tell her how much I loved her. In spirit my mother comes and helps me to understand that I have to move on and let her go but I find it hard as my heart is broken. Some Higher Being comes and takes my heart out — it's like a stone — and makes it come alive again. Then my mother comes and hugs me and puts my heart back in. We can go together now.*

At this point Kari was smiling, hugging herself and crying tears of joy. It was beautiful to see and to be part of such a profound healing process. She came out of trance with the realisation that her subconscious was not just working on releasing the cough, but it was also helping her to work on a lot of other locked-in traumas that had been holding her back and stopping her from being emotionally balanced. She was pleased that this was happening as she wanted to be the best version of herself that she could possibly be, and she knew that this regression therapy was helping her to arrive at a place of freedom.

At the start of our next session Kari told me that although she had felt good for a week or so after the last regression experience, she had started to get pictures in her mind of a past life in Africa whenever she sat and tried to relax. When she saw the pictures, she felt a lot of anger and sadness and she even had some African words coming into her head. She didn't know what they meant but she put some of the phrases into Google translate to find that they came from the Hausa language. She had never heard of Hausa before, but she found that it's an African language spoken by millions of people. One phrase which came to her over and over she put into Google translate — 'da ba la me' — to find that it means 'that is not me'.

Speaking in a foreign language in a regression session is (thankfully) an extremely rare occurrence; it's happened only twice in all of my thousands of sessions. The first time was a male client who regressed into a previous life as a Mafia boss. His whole demeanour changed as he lay in trance; his shoulders were open, his head was very upright and his face held a sneer as he spoke in Italian to me, his voice a threatening growl as he sounded as if he was giving someone an offer they couldn't refuse: 'Ravioli, pizza carbonara, Leonardo da Vinci, vorrei un tè al limone, tagliatelle'. Obviously, those were not the words he used but they sounded like them. I listened in confused bemusement. Another client started speaking Inuit in her session! Fortunately, I always keep an Inuit–English phrase book handy just in case this happens so I was able to bluff my way through. Actually, in both cases I simply asked them to talk to me in English and they immediately complied. Phew!

In Kari's case I wondered if this might happen but as soon as she closed her eyes and accessed trance she went straight into this new past life and spoke in English:

I'm an African girl around 7 years old and I'm outside a hut made of earth and straw, with my parents. I'm barefoot and I'm wearing something round my waist. I feel a little bit on edge and unsafe. There's fighting around our village and mother doesn't want father to go off hunting with the other men and leave the village unprotected. They go anyway and I'm awakened that night by the sounds of shouting and fighting. Mother picks me up and we run into the trees to hide. She's scared and she tells me to be quiet because I'm crying. There are people burning our huts. Some men find us and they take my mother. I'm frozen with fear. She's screaming as they rape and then kill her. I can't watch because it's too horrible. They take me away and make me a slave. They're from a different tribe of black people. I have to clean and make food but they treat me badly and the children bully me. I just want my mother. I keep quiet and hope they'll leave me alone. I grow up into a beautiful young woman and I don't like the boys looking at me. An older man wants me but I don't like the way he touches me. He's paid for me but I don't want to marry him. I feel hopeless and empty; there's no happiness in my life. He rapes me all the time because I don't want to have sex with him. The first time that he rapes me is awful, so painful because I'm a virgin. As I get older I to start to stand up for myself and challenge him. I stand up for the other women too. He doesn't like it and we fight but he's stronger than me. He throws me to the ground and stabs me in the throat. I'm pleased to leave that life as there was no happiness in it.

At times she had been coughing and crying, but now that she'd died in that life, she became calm again. However, it was obvious that she had moved on because a confused look came on her face and she then spoke hesitantly as if she was unsure about what she was seeing. No wonder that she was confused as it was a past life in which she was abducted by aliens:

I'm a teenage boy and I'm laid on a metal table. I don't want to be here and I'm tied down. A being is hanging up a drip which is going into my veins. I've been forced to be here to have some sort of operation. They want an organ from out of my body. They're aliens and I'm in a spaceship. They put anaesthetic into my right hand. I remember falling asleep at night and then I'm awakened by a bright light outside my bedroom window. I open the window and I'm shocked; am I awake or am I dreaming? Someone wants me to go up to them and the light takes me on board the ship. They're bigger than us, with long fingers which have round pads on the ends. They have long heads and big eyes. They take me into the operating room and they speak to me in my head. I feel scared as they take my clothes off and lay me on the table. They look into my eyes with something and then put me under. I come round after the operation and I know that they've taken one of my kidneys but when they close the wound up there's no scar. I wasn't completely knocked out during the operation but I felt no pain. They say that tomorrow when I wake up I won't remember anything and it'll be like it never happened. A needle also went into my throat and put a hard black energy into my throat. I wake up the next day at home as usual. I think they come back another time.

Kari told me that she couldn't see anything else in that life so I asked her subconscious, using her Ideo-Motor response, if the aliens had put any implants into the boy and it indicated 'yes'. It also indicated that these implants were affecting Kari in her present life, so we spent some time working to release them from her energy field. Once this was complete, she came out of trance. Kari was amazed that this little cough of hers was leading us into some highly unusual experiences!

In our next session she worked through and released three more previous lives. In the first one she was a man floating in the sea:

I'm holding onto something but I feel scared. I was cleaning the deck of a wooden boat and someone hits me from behind and pushes me into the water. I'm a sailor on board a ship and me and my friend bought a woman for money but she prefers me to him. He likes her very much and he's very angry. He hits me on the head from behind and I'm concussed. He's holding a knife to my throat and he growls "let that be a lesson to you — keep away from another man's woman" and throws me into the water. He throws a wooden barrel in the sea for me to hold onto. The water isn't too cold; I think it's off the coast of Africa. The ship keeps going and no-one knows I'm overboard. All of this because of a woman, it's stupid. I know no-one will ever find me. I'm remembering my life, being aggressive and fighting a lot. I had a lot of anger inside me. When I was a child my father beat me and hit my mother. I'm too small to help her. When I grow up, I kill my father and run away to sea. I tell my mother "now you are free but I have to go or they'll kill me". I feel sad when I think about the past. Eventually I get tired of holding onto the barrel and I slip beneath the waves and drown.

As Kari was reliving the drowning she was gasping and choking but she soon relaxed again and told me that she felt at ease. I remained silent and allowed her subconscious to take us into another life. As she began to speak she became emotional and started to shake:

I'm a woman walking along a street talking to my little girl; she's jumping and happy and dancing because we're on our way to buy her a new dress. A car suddenly comes round a corner and hits us both. It only clips me but it kills her. I'm screaming and people start running to us. I'm screaming at the driver "how could you not see her?" I'm hysterical and hitting him with my hands. She was so happy and now she's dead, just like that, in a moment. My body's gone into shock and when the ambulance arrives they give me something to calm me down. I wake up in hospital. I'm crying that I want to see my daughter but they just give me some drugs; I want to scream but I can't. I feel so guilty — I should have taken more care of her. My husband comes and he's shaking me; he blames me for her death. I feel so tense all of the time. How can I live after this? I just want to kill myself.

As she said this Kari was sobbing and choking, and this continued until she had died:

I think about cutting my wrists but I decide to drown myself. I'm in the water walking further and further in as it gets deeper. I'm so afraid but then I go under and I'm drowning. I try to hold my breath but I can't. I die and my daughter is there. She says "it's OK, we can go home now". I feel lighter. I forgive the driver and myself and I can go in peace now; I'm with my daughter again and I'm happy.

Again, Kari's body relaxed and she breathed quietly. The tears stopped and she was calm for a short time, and then her body started to jerk with anxiety:

I'm a man, a boxer, in a boxing ring. The other fighter's stronger and more aggressive than me. His eyes look as though he wants to kill me. I want to stop the fight but I can't. He hits me on the forehead and I fall to the floor; I can't stand up. I'm angry with myself; I could have pretended earlier that I was knocked out but I was afraid he'd call me a pussy. They take me hospital but I can't move because I'm in a coma. All the time I'm saying to myself "why didn't you stop it?" I'm not sure if I'll survive this as I've got a brain injury and people around me are crying. I end up being paralysed in a wheelchair. I was a strong guy and now I can't even speak. I just want them to kill me; I'm peeing and shitting myself. The other boxer is my husband in this present lifetime, he didn't want to hurt me like this but we'd argued before the fight and he was angry. A doctor sees the pain in my eyes and we talk by using my eyelids; one blink is "yes" and two blinks are "no". He asks me if I'm tired of living and I say "yes". They stop feeding me food and water. It only takes a few days. It's a relief to die. My grandmother who is in spirit comes and holds my hand and makes it easier to pass over.

Another session of releasing emotional pain was over and Kari surfaced from trance. She felt calm and happy to have let go of so much sadness, fear and anger.

At the start of our next session she told me that the cough was still reducing and that she felt much less reactive than she used to do about things that used to trigger her. She felt more secure in her marriage and her husband had noticed that she was calmer. In this session we explored another three former lives, the first one as a 4-year-old boy:

I'm walking in the countryside with my father. I'm happy but all the time I'm looking to my father as he seems quiet. I'm trying to work out what he's thinking. I want to jump around but I feel that something is wrong and it's as if he's angry. We arrive at a train station and I start to feel scared. He wants me to get on a train and sit with some other children; I don't know why I'm here. He gets off the train and leaves me with some grown-ups and the children. The train leaves and I feel scared and sad — why has he left me? We arrive at a station and we all get off together and go to a building; it's like a hospital and it's something to do with being sick from TB. It's a sanatorium and I'm there for a couple of years. I feel sad and I cry a lot as I miss my family. I start to cough blood and I'm told that I'm too sick to go home in case I pass it on to my family. I try to be brave but I get more and more sick. Eventually I go into a coma and die. An angel comes to take me and I feel a light comes into my chest to heal it when I'm in spirit. I was sad but I feel OK now.

Kari looked at ease but after a few seconds she put her hands onto her chest and started to cough. Her voice sounded anxious and panicky:

Someone's stabbing me in the chest. There's blood everywhere and I'm drowning in my own blood. An evil man is killing me. I'm a woman and I'm laid in bed. He's broke into my house. I've seen him before and he's creepy. I was at a party and he asks me if I want to dance and I laugh at him and say "no". He's angry that people are laughing at him and he wants revenge. It's like a nightmare, he suddenly appears at my door and he starts stabbing and stabbing me over and over again. I'm in shock. As I'm dying, I'm angry with myself for laughing at him; I know it was wrong to do it but I was embarrassed. I'm also thinking that you have to be careful what you say in case something bad happens. He gets away with it. I feel calm now, though I've an image of a little girl watching her parents arguing. I'm in a wheelchair and I can't walk properly. I think that my family would be better off without me because I'm handicapped.

In this new past life that she had moved into, Kari went into the character of the girl; her speech was slurred and stammering and her body twisted up in the chair as she went on:

I feel like I'm a burden as I make it hard for them. We need money but my mother can't go to work as she has to stay at home to look after me. My father doesn't love me; he has angry eyes whenever he looks at me. He's embarrassed by me; my hand works but I look stupid. One night he comes home drunk and he puts a pillow on my face and suffocates me. I hear him crying as he does it. I'm at peace now.

Kari came out of trance feeling peaceful, surprised at how many past lives she'd experienced so far, and how varied they had been. She said that they all must be coming from her subconscious as there was no way that she could imagine or make up so many stories if she tried. She knew that with every regression she was becoming more and more healed and balanced.

Our final session arrived and Kari told me that the cough had been a lot better, almost non-existent, and she had never felt so at peace and as light as she felt now. This time her subconscious had a little bit of surprise in store for us. After she had gone into trance and worked through a past life as a man who dies in the snow, her subconscious indicated that it wanted to work in the life of one of her ancestors. This was her paternal grandfather, who had sexually abused her when she was a little girl. We had already worked through and healed Kari's negative feelings of the abuse memories in an earlier session, but of course her subconscious knew that her grandfather must also have been carrying emotional baggage to have made him behave in that way. What transpired, though, as she moved into his life to experience his traumas was amazing. Unlike most of our regression sessions, in which she had been in the body of the person looking out through their eyes (in therapy terms we call this being in the first person, or associated), this time she was watching her grandfather, in a disassociated state (in the third person):

> *He's a little boy, around 7 or 8, and he's sitting alone, crying. His father's punished him for something he didn't do and it's not fair. His father's hit him with a stick on his back because he says that he's weak. His father's also hit a cat with his stick and killed it. He's a real bully. I can sense a feeling of unhappiness in his chest. He starts to close his feelings down to survive as he feels there's no-one he can trust. He begins to hurt people who he's close to. When he gets older, in his 20s, he starts to have sexual feelings for children. He starts to molest them and a part of him likes to destroy their innocence. Even though he knows that it's wrong his feelings become even darker.*

Kari now started to cough, as if trying to expel the horrible energy that she could feel in her body. She told me that she felt that the paedophile energy went back many generations, so I asked her subconscious to take her back to where it started, to the ancestor who first created this energy of paedophilia. She was quiet for a minute or two as though she was travelling back in time, and then she spoke:

I've gone a long way back through many generations. Maybe 800 years ago. There's a lot of fighting between the warriors of different tribes. I think I've gone back to Genghis Khan; he's made a woman pregnant and the child becomes a brutal man. He likes to scare people and he kills for pleasure. His mother hates him because she was raped and got pregnant with him and she brings him up badly with no love.

Kari paused in her narrative and went deeper into hypnosis. When she spoke again, she was now associated in his body and speaking in the first person. Her voice was harsh, at times almost a growl:

I just want to fight; I like to see people scared. I just take any woman I want; I don't care if they have a husband or if their husband is watching. I enjoy abusing children sexually. I feel disrespect for everything because that's how I was brought up. I remember being in the womb and my mother hating me and trying to abort me. I've never thought about this before but I'm remembering coming from a place of great love and I chose this path when I was in spirit before I was born.

This was spoken with surprise in her voice and followed by a silence, as if she (or the ancestor) were considering and processing a new insight. It was to prove to be the start of a beautiful healing process. She then continued, but her voice sounded less sure than it did before:

My mother was always stressed and not safe as there were soldiers around all of the time. I'm just an extra burden. As a baby she just pushes me away — "stop crying". I receive lots of hate from her and she hits me a lot and throws me around. I feel completely unsafe and life is just black, harsh and brutal. She just lets me cry when I'm hungry and washes me in cold water. As I grow up, I start being cruel to animals and other children, and when I grow up I think it's better to make people scared of me so that I'm safe. But it's strange. The more I think about the little baby me the more I can start to feel love for that baby. It's as though the feelings of distrust are lessening, but I can feel conflict as it's scary to let down my defences and feel these feelings. I've never felt love before for anything. How do I love? How do I love? Ah, a little baby.

I could see the turmoil that was going on inside her, as her distant ancestor started to acknowledge love instead of hatred, something he had been unable to do in his lifetime. Her lip began to pucker and tears began to stream down her face. Her arms were in front of her as if she were cradling a baby. Eventually a smile broke on her features, like the sun breaking through clouds, and she went on:

A little baby. I'm holding the little baby that was me and I've taken him away to bring him up with love; for the first time I can feel love in my heart and I'm directing the love at me, at the baby. I feel soft and loving and I don't feel that I'm a bad person anymore. I can understand why my mother was so cruel to me, it wasn't her fault, she was only reacting to her pain. I'm sending her some forgiveness, something I've never been able to do and it feels wonderful. The baby me feels safe and loved for the first time and I can feel joy and happiness flowing through me and over me and around me. It's breathtaking. I can feel all my anger dissolving away and my body is filling up with love. All the hatred in my throat is being washed away and replaced with love.

Kari lay weeping gently with a look of serene beauty on her face. She was still holding the baby in her arms as she spoke softly:

He's gone now; he's been laid to rest. I can see all the generations smiling, back through a long line of time — my father, his father, his father etc. All the way back through the generations the healing is cleansing all of them and filling them with love.

The transformation was complete. Kari's fascinating journey of healing was over. Not only was she far more emotionally balanced than she had ever been in her life, but the cough which had brought her to me in the first place was gone, and she felt a sense of freedom that flowed through every part of her body. It had been a long, tough regression process but she was finally at its end and she felt proud of her commitment to see it through. I felt proud of her too, and privileged to have been a part of it. These moments, when a client is healed and their life changed for ever, are what being a therapist is all about.

Epilogue

I sincerely hope that you have enjoyed reading about my journey as a Hypnotherapist. I am proud to be part of a profession which is dedicated to helping people to heal from their emotional, physical and spiritual wounds. It is not an easy job being a therapist, but it is an immensely rewarding one. The older I get the more I appreciate how important it is to help people heal from their emotional wounds, in order to help the world become a better place for us all. The concept that everything is interconnected is not new – Buddha spoke of it two and a half thousand years ago – but it is now becoming accepted by more and more people to be a reality, especially as quantum physics influences modern thinking in so many ways.

Therapy is a way of helping human beings become more balanced. Looking at things from the perspective of interconnectedness and the idea that none of us are truly separate from one another, as individual people become more balanced the fact that we are all connected energetically means that the world becomes more balanced. This rebalancing of human beings is an important part of helping humankind to survive the challenges that we face as a species on Mother Earth. When we are more balanced as a result of therapy, we become less reactive and more open to give and to receive love. And every client that a therapist helps to heal is one more tiny drop of love into the energy field of the collective.

The therapist's mantra:
'If I can stop one heart from breaking,
I shall not live in vain;
If I can ease one life the aching,
Or cool one pain,

Or help one fainting robin
Unto his nest again
I shall not live in vain.'
Emily Dickinson

Remember: therapy sets you free!

Biography of Steve Burgess

Steve has been a full-time Hypnotherapist in East Yorkshire, England and Norway since 1992 and in that time has completed over 15,000 one-to-one therapy sessions. He is an internationally acclaimed therapy trainer, running courses for a variety of organisations around the UK and in Norway. Steve is a former Vice-Chair of the UK Guild of Hypnotist Examiners and he is accepted as an authority on hypnotic regression, as well as being an Advanced EFT practitioner and NLP Master. He has completed many thousands of past life regressions with his clients and his books *Famous Past Lives* and *The Power of Past Life Regression* describe some of his experiences in Past Life Therapy. He has appeared on Sky One TV, GMTV and Yorkshire TV, has been regularly featured on BBC Local Radio and his work has appeared frequently in a variety of publications. He runs his own Hypnotherapy training school – Lionheart Training – and he is much in demand with online podcast and radio show hosts for his talks on hypnotherapy and past life regression. His YouTube channel '**Hypno4all**' contains a variety of Steve's free hypnotherapy recordings. Steve nowadays does all of his therapy sessions online and he has worked with clients in 26 countries around the world.

Steve's website – www.steveburgesshypnosis.com – gives more info about his work.

O-BOOKS

SPIRITUALITY

O is a symbol of the world, of oneness and unity; this eye represents knowledge and insight. We publish titles on general spirituality and living a spiritual life. We aim to inform and help you on your own journey in this life.

If you have enjoyed this book, why not tell other readers by posting a review on your preferred book site?

Recent bestsellers from O-Books are:

Heart of Tantric Sex

Diana Richardson

Revealing Eastern secrets of deep love and intimacy to Western couples.

Paperback: 978-1-90381-637-0 ebook: 978-1-84694-637-0

Crystal Prescriptions

The A-Z guide to over 1,200 symptoms and their healing crystals

Judy Hall

The first in the popular series of eight books, this handy little guide is packed as tight as a pill bottle with crystal remedies for ailments.

Paperback: 978-1-90504-740-6 ebook: 978-1-84694-629-5

Shine On

David Ditchfield and J S Jones

What if the after effects of a near-death experience were undeniable? What if a person could suddenly produce high-quality paintings of the afterlife, or if they acquired the ability to compose classical symphonies? Meet: David Ditchfield.

Paperback: 978-1-78904-365-5 ebook: 978-1-78904-366-2

The Way of Reiki

The Inner Teachings of Mikao Usui

Frans Stiene

The roadmap for deepening your understanding of the system of Reiki and rediscovering your True Self.

Paperback: 978-1-78535-665-0 ebook: 978-1-78535-744-2

You Are Not Your Thoughts

Frances Trussell

The journey to a mindful way of being, for those who want to truly know the power of mindfulness.

Paperback: 978-1-78535-816-6 ebook: 978-1-78535-817-3

The Mysteries of the Twelfth Astrological House

Fallen Angels

Carmen Turner-Schott, MSW, LISW

Everyone wants to know more about the most misunderstood house in astrology — the twelfth astrological house.

Paperback: 978-1-78099-343-0 ebook: 978-1-78099-344-7

WhatsApps from Heaven

Louise Hamlin

An account of a bereavement and the extraordinary signs — including WhatsApps — that a retired law lecturer received from her deceased husband.

Paperback: 978-1-78904-947-3 ebook: 978-1-78904-948-0

The Holistic Guide to Your Health & Wellbeing Today

Oliver Rolfe

A holistic guide to improving your complete health, both inside and out.

Paperback: 978-1-78535-392-5 ebook: 978-1-78535-393-2

Cool Sex

Diana Richardson and Wendy Doeleman

For deeply satisfying sex, the real secret is to reduce the heat, to cool down. Discover the empowerment and fulfilment of sex with loving mindfulness.

Paperback: 978-1-78904-351-8 ebook: 978-1-78904-352-5

Creating Real Happiness A to Z

Stephani Grace

Creating Real Happiness A to Z will help you understand the truth that you are not your ego (conditioned self).

Paperback: 978-1-78904-951-0 ebook: 978-1-78904-952-7

A Colourful Dose of Optimism

Jules Standish

It's time for us to look on the bright side, by boosting our mood and lifting our spirit, both in our interiors, as well as in our closet.

Paperback: 978-1-78904-927-5 ebook: 978-1-78904-928-2

www.ingramcontent.com/pod-product-compliance
Lightning Source LLC
LaVergne TN
LVHW041336190926
848399LV00037B/383